Naked and Not Ashamed

KIA POTTS

Naked and Not Ashamed

All Rights Reserved

Copyright © 2017 Kia Potts

All Rights Reserved. This book may not be reproduced, transmitted, or stored in whole or in part by any means, including graphic, electronic, or mechanical without the express written consent of the publisher except in the case of brief quotations embodied in critical articles and reviews.

Cover design: Aesthetic Ordonnance™

Celeste Publishing books may be ordered through booksellers or by contacting:

Celeste Publishing

1606 Ownby Lane

Richmond, VA, 23220

or emailing kp@iamkiapotts.com

ISBN: 978-0-9993256-0-5 (paperback)

ISBN: 978-0-9993256-1-2 (ebook)

Contents

	Introduction	5
1	Firecrackers in January	10
2	Body Love	19
3	Releasing the Weight and Embracing Love	50
4	The Launching	71
5	Contoured	79
6	The Glow Up: The Road to Becoming an Evangelist	89
7	Showing Up	106
8	Naked and Not Ashamed	110

This book is dedicated to my parents, William R. Anderson and Melody Potts Williams. Without your love, support, and encouragement; I would not be the woman I am today.

Introduction

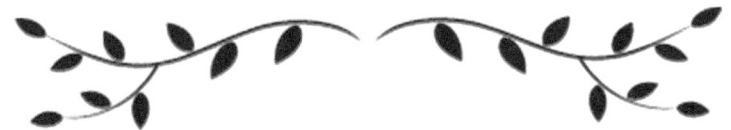

There is a beautiful story that takes place in the Book of Genesis. It begins with God putting Adam to sleep, removing a rib, and creating Eve; the first woman. Adam immediately identified with her because she was made bone of his bone and flesh of his flesh. They had an understanding that she would be his helpmeet and that they would be fruitful and multiply. But this was all under one stipulation which was simply to not eat from the tree of the knowledge of good and evil and at this time the Bible records they were both **_naked and not ashamed._** Naked, in this case, meaning innocent, baring it all, surrendering it all to God, withholding nothing, and not hiding anything. Just living in peace, and on one accord, in the Garden of Eden.

6 Naked and Not Ashamed

If you are reading this book, chances are, you can relate to a time of innocence where you were not aware of trials and tribulations. You were not aware of heartbreak, pain, abuse, or evil. All you knew was simply how to live in this world with the provision God gave you. Until you were exposed to a lie or deceived, much like how Eve was misguided.

You see, it wasn't until the seed of doubt was placed in her that she began to question what God said. The serpent's assignment in the garden was to try to make her unsure of who and whose she was and to make her feel as though she was not enough. Once these thoughts of insecurity and uncertainty took root in Eve, the perfect environment for confusion was then cultivated enough for her to make a decision based on what she thought she was lacking. She made a decision based off of ungodly counsel to disobey God and partook in eating from the forbidden tree, the very thing God told her and Adam not to touch.

Many of us are guilty of this. If we are honest, we continue to be active participants in our own disobedience *(see the chapter titled Contoured)*. When Adam and Eve willingly ate from the forbidden tree, there was an immediate transformation that took place. They became aware of the difference between good and evil. The definition of their nakedness changed.

There are various definitions of nakedness. There is ***arowm***, which is *an innocent form of nakedness*; ***eyrom***, which is *an exposing form of nakedness*; and then there is ***ervah***, which is *a shameful or indecent nakedness*. They went from having a form of innocent nakedness to being exposed, and thus, feeling shame from that exposure upon discovering that God was not pleased with their decisions. Adam and Eve's nakedness, or innocence, was perverted to shame.

How do we know this? The Bible states that they tried to cover themselves with fig leaves once they realized they were not covered. In other words, once they realized that their sin was exposed they no longer felt a sense of innocence. So now you have this couple who, at first, were living free. They had no worries in life; did not carry guilt, did not know what insecurity or low self-esteem was; not to mention doubt. And now they were living in an oppressed state. The very thing they believed would bring them closer to God or make them "like little gods", actually ended up putting a wedge in their relationship with Him. What they were created to do and achieve now required them to work for it. For Adam, he would have to sweat from his brow to eat *(Genesis 3:18)* and for Eve there would be a constant battle between her, the serpent, and her and Adam's offspring *(Genesis 3:15)*.

The same applies for us today. We were all created for an assignment on this Earth, but for some of us, somewhere we got misguided in our own Garden of Eden and experienced the heartbreaking and life changing moment, or moments, of shame. The Garden of Eden represents when we were at total oneness with God, a moment of Glory we encountered with Him where there was peace. From the beginning we were forbidden to eat from the tree of knowledge of good and evil because God knew it would be too much for us to handle. Some of you may have once had an innocence about you that caused you to live life freely, not letting fear or past experiences hold you back. Not being bitter, angry, or cynical. Then you went through a painful breakup, experienced an abusive relationship, a divorce, someone you loved — without warning — abandoned you, or someone you were close to died. Maybe you were molested or sexually assaulted, or you have experienced so many disappointments in life that you are afraid to live. *I get it!* Life can be hard. The journey while accomplishing the assignment is not always clear but we know we have a purpose.

This book is for those who have an idea of their purpose and maybe lost their way, lost confidence, or; are living their purpose and pursuing it, yet still carrying some luggage from a previous journey which is slowing down the progress of moving forward.

I know all about knowing you have a bigger purpose in life but still not living to your full potential in God. I always knew God wanted me to be someone impactful and that I was different but I did not understand how until now. For years I was held back by things from my childhood and past that perverted my confidence and free spirit to feelings of shame, insecurity, and low self-esteem. I knew in order to get back to my true innocence or identity it would require me healing from my past and removing any seeds of doubt that were planted in my spirit. This book is a memoir inspired by God. I'm just the vessel He chose to live and write the story. He gets all the glory!

I hope my testimony and everything I have been through in life thus far will shine light on those dark areas of your life and bring forth healing. This book is designed to provoke transformation and reformation in your life. This is my truth. This is how I went from hiding my truth to being **Naked and Not Ashamed.**

Be inspired.

1

Firecrackers in January

Bright colors, sparkles, excitement, joy...this described my demeanor as a child. I was always positive and always saw the good in every situation or person. I had no experience of hatred or violence. I could not even imagine that people could do bad things, until one night I awakened to the sound of *"firecrackers"*.

I was so excited to see the fireworks, I did not care that they had disrupted my sleep. I ran to my mother's room and I said, "Mom, someone is lighting fireworks outside!"

Before I could crack the blinds open to look she anxiously yelled, "GET DOWN!"

I was confused. "Why can't I see the fireworks!?" I exclaimed.

Firecrackers in January   11

She said, "Because those are not firecrackers, those are gunshots!!!"

Immediately, feelings of fear and danger resided in me. My world as I knew it would forever be changed. That's the moment my anxiety began and my innocence and optimistic view of the world ended as I repeatedly heard ripples of shots being fired. It sounded like a machine gun and when the bullets ran out, they reloaded and more shots were fired.

It seemed like it would never end. With every bullet that was fired off it felt like a piece of my innocence went with them. Even after they stopped shooting, the sounds in my head remained, "Pow, Pow, Pow!" I wanted to disappear but I couldn't. This was my reality now. The place of peace and safety as I knew it was forever gone.

Once the gunfire stopped there was more noise to follow. The sounds of screams, terror, and heartbreak belted out all at once. "No! No! No! Nooooo!" I couldn't believe what I was hearing. I couldn't believe this was happening. Then there were lights and sirens as the police and ambulance made their entrance into the parking lot. Their arrival prompted neighbors to feel secure enough to peep through their doors. As the night unfolded, my mom broke the news that my next door neighbor had been shot and killed.

I was beside myself with not knowing how to process everything that had just happened. How can the same guy I saw earlier and knew be dead? How could they kill him in such a horrible way? How could they unload

12 Naked and Not Ashamed

the gun on him and then reload to unload again? How could a person take another person's life?

I was nine years old trying to make sense of a senseless violent crime. I wanted so badly for the sounds I heard to be firecrackers in January. I wanted to see the beautiful dances of sparkles as the flames were dispersed into the sky. I wanted to be wowed and amazed by the dance of the colors that illuminated the sky. Instead, a horrible feeling of doom and gloom entered into my environment. The perspective in which I once saw the world would never be the same.

I don't think I got any sleep that night and the next day I had to go to school as if everything was normal. I had to pretend that I did not have to step over the blood stains on the sidewalk or as if I was not traumatized by what my ears and imagination had witnessed. I began to process it the best way I knew how and that was to suppress my emotions. Why? Everyone else around me seemed to cope just fine. They were laughing, joking, playing and eating like nothing ever happened. Perhaps they did not experience what I experienced. Perhaps they did not hear what I heard.

There were no resources available to help me deal with the post-traumatic stress disorder symptoms I experienced from hearing the sounds of murder. My new normal became me being absolutely terrified at anything that remotely resembled or sounded like a gunshot. The most puzzling thing was that it seemed like I was the only one that was internalizing what had happened. It was as if everyone else moved on and I was stuck in time with the events replaying over and over again in my head. Why weren't my friends as shocked as I was? How were they handling it so well? I had so many questions but no answers. No one to explain anything and nobody to fully articulate the why and the how. All that was around me was confusion, grief, and weariness.

As I began my coping journey, anxiety and fear became my best friends. I would depend on anxiety to try and figure out what was going to happen next. I was so thrown off by the event and that everything was out of my control that I would depend on fear to control my life. To a nine year old this seemed logical. That way I would at least expect the worst and not be so caught off guard. I could not control my environment or the neighborhood. No matter how much I begged my mom to move, the reality was that she did not have the resources to do so.

At this point, I began to despise my community. Even worse, I would compare my upbringing to those of the kids I went to school with; who lived in nice houses, had both parents and did not have to worry about witnessing a violent crime.

Growing up in a single parent household, I just hated everything about my life. Wanting so badly to get out, but could not. There is nothing worse in life than feeling trapped and stuck in an overly toxic environment. What options did I have, one might ask? Absolutely none. My only escape was sleepovers at my friend's houses, in their nice neighborhoods, with their perfectly manicured lawns. I used to think, 'Wow, it must feel good to come home and not feel afraid, and to be in a peaceful and quiet area.'

At that age, I had an understanding of God, but I was not mature enough spiritually to know how to turn to Him for prayer and peace. I had no idea how to articulate and express how I was feeling. However, my body had a way of responding for me. I began to develop ulcers in my mouth. They were big and painful. My mom took me to the dentist to see what could be done but to no avail. The dentist could only recommend an oral pain reliever for comfort and, unfortunately, there was really nothing he could do about it. Surprisingly, he confirmed the cause of these ulcers was stress.

Can you believe it? At nine years old I was stressed. Stressed to the point that it begin to affect me physically. I was living in an environment that I did not deem safe while simultaneously trying to process everything that had happened. To say that I was unhappy would be an understatement. I was so embarrassed and ashamed of where I lived. Some teachers even had a made up mind about how the students from my neighborhood would behave and perform academically. So when I told them where I lived they were appalled. Why? Because I was a straight A student and mild mannered. I guess you could say I was the exception to the status quo.

I wanted everything about my life to change. Why couldn't I grow up in a nice quiet neighborhood? At least then I would not have to deal with trying to be a normal 9 year old. In hindsight I realized that when you experience something as horrific as hearing someone get murdered, you develop a new normal. A normal where you learn how to cope the best you know how without treatment, just trying to survive.

I do not believe in the philosophy that 'time heals all wounds' but rather what you do in that time determines how well you heal. Unfortunately, my survival method was to suppress my feelings and internalize my emotions. I did not express them even if someone asked me if something was wrong. My plan was to pretend as though I did not feel anything. I realized I had a long ways to go before I could go off to college, graduate, get a career and make enough money to control my environment and safety. So until then, I had to guard my emotions and what I felt. I trained myself to do this by constantly practicing holding back tears and suppressing my true emotions. I hated to cry in front of people and showing any sign of what I thought was weakness.

My coping strategies of pretending not to feel anything only treated the symptoms but did not fully get to the root of the issues and unhappiness. Eventually my method of coping could no longer keep the symptoms at rest and my best friends fear and anxiety; and my acquaintance, which was post-traumatic stress; would want to hang out with me from time to time. It was usually when my environment seemed unsafe to me such as people fighting, yelling or any type of hostile situation or when I felt like I had no control over a situation. My best friends and acquaintance were faithfully by my side. It was not until I embarked on a spiritual journey that I truly began to let them go.

16 Naked and Not Ashamed

We all have scars and wounds that on the outside may seem completely healed, but it is not until we get below the surface level that we began to recognize that there still may be some scar tissue (residue) present. We may discover that the wound may still have some tender spots depending on weather conditions or other factors. That maybe it did not quite heal properly because it was not treated or cared for correctly during its most vulnerable phases.

I wish I could tell you that my healing treatments worked and that I was not affected at all by the environment I grew up in, but that would be a lie. My truth is at the time no one fully understood what I was battling...not my family, my friends and not even me! Only God knew. I did not realize how much that dreadful night affected me until at a meeting at work we were asked to think of a childhood experience that changed us forever. Immediately, the shooting was brought to my memory. I believe this was God's way of reminding me that I needed to talk about it. So with a trembling and shaky voice, fighting back tears, I told my co-workers about my experience.

For a moment, I felt liberated and that a weight had lifted. They could not believe it. Some even made comments like, "I couldn't imagine!" This started the healing process because it was the first time other people had validated the fact that I had every right to feel what I felt. This was important because when you grow up in a community like I did, the motto was to; keep it moving, don't look like a punk, and do what you have to do to survive. As I was talking about it, I knew I had to continue to share my experience with others.

Expressing and sharing what you have been through not only helps others but it helps you. It is an essential part of the healing process. If I had known then what I know now, I would have definitely asked my mom if I could talk to a counselor. It is unfortunate that so many people do not believe in seeking help or talking to someone, African Americans especially.

As an African American woman, I was raised to be strong and self-sufficient so I even developed a sense of pride and had a notion that only weak people needed those types of things. However, I now realize it takes a very strong and mature person to recognize that when they are wounded it is ok to ask for help.

We were never meant to carry our burdens alone. **Iron sharpens iron.** God is the ultimate source and He sends people as resources in our lives. Resources may include therapy, spiritual counseling, and so many other methods. If you have experienced something traumatic, do not think you have to hide or be embarrassed about it. Get the help you need so you can be free from whatever is holding you back.

I honestly believe I spent years coping the best way I knew how with undiagnosed post-traumatic stress disorder and anxiety. After learning how to function with these disorders for so long, they become a part of my life thus creating a new normal. I thought it was my job to worry, to not have peace, and to be afraid all of the time. It was not until later in my adult life when I began to work on myself and had a spiritual awakening, that I began to heal. Faith without works is dead so I began going to therapy as well as attend church. My prayer life strengthened and my relationship with God strengthened. As my relationship with God strengthened I began to understand my purpose clearly. With that understanding, more of that fear, anxiety, and worry began to subside as I knew I still had more work to do on this Earth. I knew God wanted to use me to help others. Slowly but surely God was restoring everything that was lost, damaged and broken from the past.

2

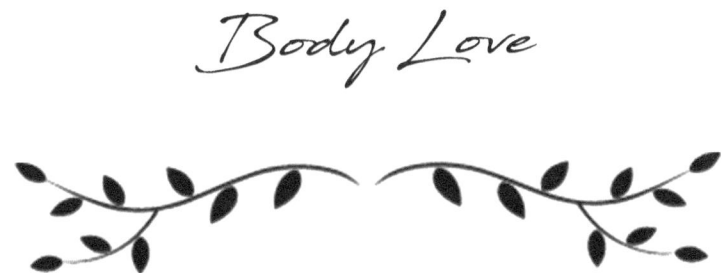

A city on a hill cannot be hidden, if they're looking for You let them find You in me.

Matthew 10:29-31, "Are not two sparrows sold for a penny? And not one of them will fall to the ground apart from your Father. But even the hairs of your head are all numbered. Fear not, therefore; you are of more value than many sparrows"

I wish I had the scripture, *Matthew 10:29-31*, hidden in my heart. This would have given me the strength I needed at the time. There were some many times as an adolescent and teenager where I wanted to hide and not be seen at all.

As a little girl I always felt beautiful because I had a mother who would always affirm me. She also took the time to nurture me by doing many acts of service for me such as taking care of my hair (I had long beautiful waist length hair by the age of eight). She made sure I was well dressed and looked presentable. Strangers would approach her and say, "You have a beautiful little girl." I didn't fully comprehend what that meant but I knew it was something positive because my mom would tell me to say thank you. So my identity in beauty came from what I heard from other people and my mom's love towards me. Relying on other's opinion, I never developed my own understanding or definition of beauty at a young age.

My mom would always encourage me to challenge myself. She once entered me into a radio station dance contest. I was somewhat shy around strangers and didn't want to do it, but her love allowed me to freely engage in activities beyond my comfort zone. It wasn't until I was going through the metamorphosis of puberty that I began to question my looks, self-image, and idea of beauty.

I began to develop pretty early, about the age 11, I would say. By the time I was 14, I had the figure of a woman, yet still the mindset and innocence of a child. This made it difficult for me to comprehend all the attention that came with having a shapely figure and by shapely figure I mean hips, thighs, a butt, and chest. I was very curvy for my age and with that came a lot of unwanted sexual advances from males that were my peers as well as adult men.

I always wondered why some people were outgoing and why some people were more reserved and shy. I wanted so badly to be more outgoing instead of being the quiet girl. I did not understand why I did not like attention or being the center of attention while some people loved it, it made me uncomfortable. I used to dislike being this way but in retrospect, I thank God my demeanor was as such because while others may have thrived off of or felt flattered by being hit on, it only repulsed me and sometimes frightened me. It was never affirming to me to hear explicit "catcalls" or to have a boy touch me inappropriately. Even in my youth, I knew it was unhealthy behavior so I never mistook it for love or being liked.

I began to get sexually harassed at the age of eleven. Only back then, if it was the kids doing it, it wasn't considered sexual harassment. People brushed it off as "boys being boys." I did not realize how much attention my body attracted until an incident occurred at a summer camp I was attending.

It was a hot summer and we were all thrilled about being out of school. I looked forward to attending my annual summer camp where I would be able to reconnect with all my friends from last year and we could enjoy playing tennis, basketball, taking field trips, and just having the fun that comes with being a kid. I could not wait to get into the pool because I also loved swimming.

Swimming was the highlight of the day. It was the number one activity that I enjoyed. In the water I felt free, relaxed, and rejuvenated. I could do flips in the water, splash, handstands, float, and do all the fun things kids like to do in the pool. Swimming was an activity I thoroughly enjoyed and it was soooooo exciting to me, but it quickly became an activity I could no longer enjoy that summer.

I remember the swim suit I was wearing. It was a lovely blue and white two piece that my mom bought from New York for me. I loved it! It was stylish yet functional. I eagerly changed into my two piece in the locker room because I was so excited to get into the pool. I could smell the chlorine and hear the splashes and laughter of those already enjoying their swim time. Fun time in the pool was the best part about summer camp. There were so many things I could do in the pool that I couldn't on land. I already envisioned me doing flips and handstands. Again, I felt so free!

As I began to approach the pool, I saw some of the boys smiling and grinning. They had mischievous looks on their faces as if they were up to no good and was about to execute a well devised plan. They were definitely plotting.

As soon as I entered the pool, they began to execute their plan of attack. Unfortunately, the victim was yours truly. One would go under the water to try and pull down my bikini bottoms or grab my behind. The other boys would try to unsnap my bathing suit top or touch my breasts. All that was running through my mind was that 'I cannot let them win. They will not get the satisfaction of fulfilling their conquest of violating and humiliating me,' but no matter how much I would fight back and attempt to kick them in their private area, they would still keep pursuing me. It was as if the harder I fought the more they enjoyed it.

I remember being so disgusted by the mischievous looks on their faces when they were successful at grabbing my butt or touching breasts. I was extremely disturbed and angry by this. I had a range of emotions, which resulted in my best solution at the time for a response to my violation, and that was to fight back. But, it did not matter how hard or frequent I hit them because they had accomplished their goal.

That day will forever be in my memory. I will never forget how I felt. It was as if they had taken away my peace, my happiness, my innocence. I felt like it was my fault or that I did something wrong. Maybe if I was mean, wasn't so quiet, shy, and timid they would not have bothered me. Maybe if I wasn't so developed for my age they would have not even looked at me. I felt defeated, I felt weak, and I felt like they had won and had taken a part of me with them. That day they took my dignity, my self-esteem, my sense of self-worth, my confidence (what little I had at that age), and my innocence. I was too embarrassed and ashamed to tell any of the camp counselors and the ones that did witness it just ignored what was happening or did not take action. I felt like I was in a battle all on my own. That no one understood my pain, my embarrassment, humiliation, and my shame.

After the pool activity was over no one came to me and talked to me about what I had experienced. It was as if nothing happened and that it was ok and normal for those boys to have behaved that way. I felt awkward and I did not feel comfortable discussing it with the camp counselors there; especially the male ones. How could I trust any males after that? Even worse, how could I explain to them the event that occurred? That would require me to relive the experience in my head, and that was too painful and embarrassing to endure. So I buried it to cope and pretended that it did not bother me so much.

    I have always had a close relationship with my mother. Ever since I could remember she would always say, "If anyone ever touches you inappropriately please tell me. Don't be afraid to come to me because you can come to me about anything."

    I remembered these words as they were embedded in me and that night I felt compelled to tell my mom, so I did. The next day she told the counselors, but it did not make a difference. The counselors were not equipped nor trained to handle a problem of this nature. A fist fight they could deal with; a little horse play or even bullying; but when it came to sexual assault no one wanted to touch it and as a result nothing changed.

    The boys would still try me and eventually, I had to stop swimming. I felt like that would be the only solution to the problem, but it was not. The boys would still try to grab my butt, touch my breast, and sexually assault me when no one was watching outside of the pool. I did not understand why other girls at the camp did not have this problem. Why was I the only one getting picked on? Was it because I was seemingly shy and timid? Was I too quiet? Or was it the fact that I did not like a lot of attention that made me appear weak and made me an easy target to become a prey to predators?

Again, I thank God I was repulsed by it and did not respond to it in a way that was pleasing to man because when you invite that type of attention into your life, you open the door to so many things such as lust and perversion. Even at that age I knew that was a path I did not want to entertain. Ironic enough, the attention still had an effect on me, the extreme opposite effect.

I begin to internalize everything and blamed myself.

I would reason in my mind, *If I didn't have this body type, then I wouldn't have this problem* or *If I was skinny they wouldn't bother me.*

This was the deception that was planted in my head that would make the journey to having a healthy self-image a long and hard one.

It seemed like the older I got, the worse the aggressiveness and lustful stares became. It was Labor Day weekend and my mom and stepdad at the time (who was from Trinidad) decided to take a spontaneous trip to Brooklyn, New York for the annual Labor Day weekend parade. I was excited, I thought this would be my first trip to New York. At the time I was thirteen. I remember all the things I learned, when I was younger, about the "Big Apple" by watching movies set in New York City. I would always hear stories from other people who traveled there about how fun and fascinating it was; the great fashions, the excitement, the hustle and bustle, the food, the buildings, the lights, the Statue of

26 Naked and Not Ashamed

Liberty, the Empire State Building, and the celebrities they would see. I would always admire Times Square from the New Year's Eve shows that came on television and thought, 'Wow, what an amazing place!'

As a kid growing up, so many of the things I saw on television shows seemed abstract and like I would never have the opportunity to visit those places. So when they told us we were going to New York, it was like a dream come true. I thought, 'Wow!!!! I'm going to get to visit the Empire State Building, The Statue of Liberty, go see a Broadway show, and all the other fun touristy things kids love to do.' I loved to travel and lived for a new adventure.

As we arrived in New York in the wee hours of the morning, the scene was a little different than I had imagined. This was not the New York I saw on television. I did not see any of the tourist sites only rows of town houses. I did not get to experience any of the things I wanted to experience, but what I did experience was something that was truly unforgettable.

My idea of a parade was floats, big balloons, and marching bands. However, nothing could prepare me for the Caribbean Labor Day Parade experience (it was definitely not like any other parade I had ever attended). Well maybe the ride on the train to get to Flatbush Avenue. It was a hot summer day and the train was packed to capacity. So much so that we had to wait sometimes for another train to come because we could not fit anywhere. I mean, there were crowds of people dressed in their festive costumes with masks and face paintings.

When we reached our destination, the streets were filled and flooded with people from all different walks of life. On top of experiencing culture shock, it was difficult to maneuver through the crowd and because there was music playing and it was a party atmosphere some people felt they had the privilege to dance with you any kind of way. There were men of all ages from middle age to really old trying to dance behind me. They would just jump behind me and grind on me. It was difficult to get away from it because we were packed like sardines on the street. The fact that I was not engaging in any movement with them, I thought, was a clear indicator that I did not want to dance with them let alone want them to touch me at all. My mom did not realize what was going on as she was enjoying the festivities.

Suddenly, I began to get a flashback of the events that took place in the pool at summer camp and it was not until I began to cry and have a panic attack that she realized what was happening. I was terrified, I had never experienced this before. The men were aggressive and would pull me close to them. I felt helpless. Like something was wrong with me and no one understood because everyone else seemed to enjoy the close dancing. They may have assumed I was older because of my figure but in my mind that was still no excuse for them to force themselves into my space. After that experience, I just wanted to leave New York all together. I wanted to quickly leave the area of the parade. I was being harassed by men who looked old enough to be my grandfather. It was like being in that pool all over again. I felt helpless, afraid and ignored.

That summer camp experience really changed my life. Not only did I become self-conscious and hypervigilant (so much to the point that it triggered a spirit of low self-esteem and whenever I was in the presence of a teenager or adult male I would not want to walk in front of them for fear of being grabbed or gawked upon), but there was an ungodly impartation that occurred the day I was sexually assaulted which opened the door for me to experience more sexual harassment and uncomfortable situations, especially when it came to adult men. They would go out of their way to look at me not in a way of admiration but with eyes of lust. With each penetrating look, I felt as though they were undressing me and I would feel naked. Not in a way that was empowering or liberating, but more so that of a disposition that yielded shame and made me want to hide even when I was fully clothed.

I was not aware of this until one afternoon my mom and I decided to take a trip to Walmart. We were walking towards the entrance, and me being the naive young lady I was, I did not even notice the man that had purposely slowed down his steady pace. His plan was to slow down so he could get a good look at my backside once I passed by.

My mother being the insightful and observant, as well as protective, mother that she was (and still is) whispered in my ear, "That man is waiting for us to walk by so he can look at you."

In other words, he was trying to get a good look at my body. I was a little taken aback and immediately my best friends fear and anxiety returned and I did not know what to do. I certainly did not want to give him such satisfaction especially when he was being so obvious. I did not want to feel cheap and humiliated all over again.

My mom came up with a plan and told me, "When we get to him turn around and walk backwards."

I followed her orders. The man tried to play it off as though he had other intentions but my mom yelled at him, "She's only 14!!!"

Although there was a little victory in this moment, I knew that there would probably be many more instances such as this or many that had already occurred and I never even realized it. Even though I was not touched by the man, there was still a sense of violation I experienced. I felt singled out and embarrassed at the fact that a simple trip to Walmart turned into a life lesson.

My very first job was also my very first experience of being harassed at work. I was 14 and I was excited to be working and making my own money. I got paid about $125.00 every two weeks. With no bills to pay and no responsibilities, that was a lot of money for a 14 year old. I liked going to work and meeting new people, until some of the teenage boys that worked there got a little too friendly. They would act as though they accidently bumped into me or mistakenly grazed my butt or the side of my breast. I would react the only way I knew

30 Naked and Not Ashamed

how and that was by fighting back. Once again, this did nothing, they would just laugh and do it again. I was too embarrassed to tell my boss who was also a man. I did not know how he would receive it and if I could trust him. This behavior continued for a while with multiple guys that worked there. There was one guy who worked there with his girlfriend and every time she was not around he would constantly proposition me to sleep with him and go on and on about how great in bed he was. This was wrong on so many levels. I was so disgusted; one, by the fact that he had the audacity to approach me in that way and he thought I would be receptive to that; and two, that he had no respect or regard toward his girlfriend. I did not have the courage to tell my manager or anyone for that manner. It was again too embarrassing explaining and putting into words what was happening. It was not until a lady that worked there witnessed someone sexually harassing me that it was reported. Management took what happened very seriously and there were warnings given. I did not have any issues at work after that, but I still had issues with my body.

    These events perpetuated my hatred toward my body even more. I tried to wear clothes that would hide my hips and butt and when I did wear clothes that showed my curves or legs, I felt so uncomfortable. I recalled on many occasions staring in the mirror and feeling so ugly. I hated my body. I can recollect taking my hands and placing them on each side of my hips and trying to push my hips in. It was not the most rational hour of my life but I just wanted to picture myself without them. I thought if I could just get rid of them I would feel and look so much better. I did not understand why this was happening to me all the time and I didn't like it. It was as if I was being undressed with my clothes on and I could not do anything about it and I was most certainly not provoking it. I began to develop an anxiety about being in public because I never knew what loud or lewd remarks would be expressed by men, who would follow me or worse who would try to touch me.

It took me so long to get ready in the mornings because I was so uncomfortable with anything that showed any of my womanly curves. It didn't dawn on me that this still affected me as an adult until I would put so much effort into getting ready for church.

I did not want to attract lustful spirits and I did not want people assuming I was promiscuous because of how my clothes fit my body. Getting ready for church was a stressful event. It took my best friend to tell me that because my body was curvy clothes just fit me differently. She went on to say that it was not a bad thing or it did not mean I was trying to attract attention.

She was really upfront with me and said, "Look, you got a butt and hips, so your clothes are going to fit you differently, that's all."

Thank God for best friends that know how to quickly put things in perspective for you. She said that it's nothing to be ashamed of...and if anybody has an issue with it, it's their problem. I needed to hear those words. I needed to be validated and liberated from someone I knew without a doubt had my best interest at heart.

My body issues affected the activities I participated in as well. I wanted so badly to be on the gymnastics team in middle school. It wasn't the nervousness of tryouts that deterred my decision of joining, nor the fear of being rejected, but the fact that I would have to wear a leotard in front of so many people was the deciding factor on not auditioning for the team. I did not want people looking at me in something that would reveal so much of my body. I was afraid I was going to experience the same reactions that I had experienced at the swimming pool and that was a memory I wanted to erase all together.

I was in bondage and this bondage hindered me from doing the activities that I loved. It was difficult to express to people who asked me, why are you not on the gymnastics team or why are you not swimming. Not many thirteen year olds would understand my dilemma and I couldn't quite put language to what I was dealing with myself. I was too embarrassed and ashamed to discuss what had happen to me in the pool that day and what was continuing to happen from the time I began to develop.

The sexual harassment and assault became so frequent that eventually it became normal for me...so much so I assumed every female encountered these types of experiences.

Throughout my adolescent and teenage years, I tried to overcome my battles. I was a cheerleader throughout grade school. I also studied dance in high school. Being a cheerleader and a dancer helped me to be comfortable with being in front of people and not to be so self-conscious. I still had my moments of self-loathing. I vividly remember looking at my reflection in the mirror while I had on my cheerleading outfit or leotard. As I mentioned before, I pressed the sides of my skirt against my hips to see how I would look if I didn't have my curves. I would do this often. I thought, if I could just not have so much hips, I would feel better about my body. It also did not help that I had some family members who felt the need to comment on my shape and body.

They would constantly say, "You better watch that figure, you don't want gain any weight, you are alright at that size but just don't get any bigger."

Huh? What? This was not encouraging at all to a teenager who already had body image issues. Their comments just added more pressure and anxiety to my body/weight issues. These were constant seeds, planted into my head by some family members that did not make me feel better about myself at all. Only more aware of my flaws.

I could not understand how some people would complement me on my body and others would try to, in so many words, say I was on the borderline of being fat. I felt so insecure about my body and I was always uncomfortable.

It was not until now that I realized that people who try to make other people feel uncomfortable about themselves are more than likely also uncomfortable with their own image and they will reflect those insecurities they have about themselves onto you. I was young and not wise enough to know this. Therefore, I took every commentary from people to heart and ultimately it only increased the insecurities I had of my own.

This is where people, especially women, need to realize that we cannot search for our identity in others. We cannot look to others for confirmation or to make us feel beautiful about ourselves, our bodies, or anything else. You are the one that has to live in your body so only you can decide whether you are comfortable in it or not. People will always try to find something to pick apart about you, but you have to get to the point where you love your body no matter what and can look in the mirror and see imperfections, assets, and scars and still say that you love yourself. You cannot allow people to rip you apart because then you give them the power to make you feel less than when really, they are the ones unhappy with the reflection that appears in the mirror.

When I look back at my high school photos, there was nothing wrong with my size. I was just shaped differently and had curves. Having curves does not mean that you are fat, it is simply how you are structured. Because my figure was such a "concern" to some of the women in my family; and I would hang on to their every word, opinions, and comments about my body and because I wanted their approval; I would go on the unhealthiest diets they would recommend.

One diet consisted of a Slimfast for breakfast, a Slimfast for lunch, and a lean cuisine for dinner. This was starvation for me. I was a very active teenager involved in cheerleading and dance so this amount of food was not enough calories to even sustain a 5 minute walk let alone a two hour game or a ninety minute dance class. I could not figure out why I was so hungry and I thought I must just be greedy so I would endure it. I liked the results and the praise I would get from family members when they saw I was "coming down" in size. After all, I was looking for affirmation and approval. However, after a while I would just throw in the towel and eat what I wanted.

When I studied dance in high school, I knew in order for me to look in the mirror, I had to suppress. Not really heal from, but suppress my body image issues. In dance class, we had to wear leotards and tights. Remember how this was a fear of mine in middle school. I loved dance so much, I did what I needed to do to cope and that was pretend as though it did not bother me.

To heighten the intensity of the experience, we had mirrors all over the studio. It was bad enough that I had to be in front of people in this attire, but I also had to see myself in it. I constantly had to change in front of other girls as well, which was uncomfortable for me because I did not want them to see my body and make comments about it. Don't get me wrong, there were some days where I did appreciate my body. Those days were usually if I had starved myself for three days and thought I had lost a significant amount of weight. It was all in my head. It was always hard because there was no category for me. The skinny girls were obviously skinny, the chubby girls were obviously chubby and then there was me. I had a flat stomach, small torso, but big legs and thighs, hips and a butt. 'Where do I fit in?' I would always wonder. I would constantly compare my body to my fellow dance class mates. I thought of myself as a horrible dancer because I felt if I were smaller, my dance moves would look better. I was battling internally with this all throughout high school.

The ironic part was no one really teased me about my body. Some people, male and female, were actually very complimentary.

I remember one prom I wore a certain dress and everyone was like, "Only you could have worn that dress because of your body." I thought wow there are people that actually appreciate my shape!

Although I was flattered by the compliments, I was not able to fully take them in or accept what I was hearing because to me my body was not my ideal image of beauty. I wanted to be slim and not curvy. I hated my butt and my big legs. Things that some the smaller girls longed for (at least in my circle), I rejected.

I learned a lot of lessons from comparing myself to others. The most important one is that under no circumstances should any woman compare herself to another woman. We are all fearfully and wonderfully made (Psalm 139:14). That means when we were created, God gave each of us a specific and unique design. Everything God does is purposeful and He was intentional in His creation of us. God does not make mistakes but He makes masterpieces. We are all a masterpiece in His big plan. You may not be deemed perfect by the world but All that is good and perfect comes from Him (James 1:17).

In my years of struggling with my self-esteem and body image, I have learned that comparing myself to others only sparks self-hatred and does not promote self-love. There is a difference between celebrating a way another person looks and feeling unworthy because you do not have the same physique. The very same thing you are complaining about regarding your body, another person probably aspires to have. You do not know that other person's story, she may be struggling with her own body image. There are no perfect people and that is why we cannot get so wrapped up in looking like models, actresses, musicians, or your favorite celebrity. We have to be content with all of our flaws, marks, and imperfections. I am an advocate for striving to grow and improve yourself, however; coveting someone's look can spark a seed of envy and can lead to low self-esteem.

We may begin to wonder, how is it that this person is shaped like this and I am not? How can I get my body to look like theirs? You have to change your mindset and attitude. Instead of asking the how and why you can practice thanking your body. Appreciate yourself so when others do you can fully embrace their compliments.

> ***Romans 12:1,*** *I beseech you therefore, brethren, by the mercies of God, that you present your bodies a living sacrifice, holy, acceptable to God, which is your reasonable service.*

Self-hatred can manifest itself in many ways. It can make one feel like they will never be desired or wanted. It can make one feel as though they are a disgrace to others. It can make one stop eating or over eat. It can make one make bad decisions and behave in an uncharacteristic manner. For me it made me love, love, love food and I often over ate a lot because I suppressed my emotions and feelings and would try to fill it with food. I was the one at Thanksgiving that would go back for thirds, fourths and fifths. I also loved and still love sweets (guilty pleasure).

   I remember one Valentine's Day my mom bought my brother, herself, and me a box of chocolates. I enjoyed the chocolates and quickly devoured mine as if I had not eaten in months. As fast as I opened the box was just as fast as I ate them. Once I was finish the feeling of them not being there anymore was disappointing and it saddened me. I wanted that feeling of satisfaction back. I wanted that burst of euphoric feeling I felt when I tasted the goodness and richness of the sweet chocolate. So without any regard to anyone else, I also ate my mom and my brother's chocolates. I did not care about the fact that I was being selfish or greedy, I just wanted to feel good and if that meant eating someone else's chocolates, then so be it. Having this attitude only led to an unhealthy relationship with food.

   Whenever there was food and an abundance of it, it was not a good thing for me. My greedy spirit would set in and I would want to devour everything in sight. Especially if it was free. I perceived it as my duty not to let free food go to waste. My mind was all distorted and messed up. I thought the more I filled up the more satisfaction I would receive. Thank God for deliverance! In retrospect, I learned as long as you are filling yourself with temporary fixes, you are only going to yield temporary results. When you eat that meal to fill an emotional void you are going to yield a temporary emotional response.

The feeling of gratification from eating food and desserts was only a short moment of pleasure but the effects it had on my body yielded weight gain and a low self-image.

I was a sensitive child and in the neighborhood I grew up in, it was not cool to be this way. So I learned how to hide my emotions. Food became my refuge. It was my stronghold and it gave me comfort. This did not become a problem until I got older and began to gain weight. My weight was 138 pounds my freshman year in college and by the time I graduated, I had skyrocketed up to 195 pounds. Although the weight gain did not affect the opposite sex from showing me attention, it did however make me have even more issues with my body. So much to the point I became even more self-conscious. I became even more uncomfortable in my own skin.

The weight gain took a toll on me and I was in a constant battle with my mind. I would tell myself you need to be content this way because you are never going to be smaller again, this is it for you. Even now, it is hard to believe I lied to myself so much. Deep down in my spirit, I knew it did not sit with me well to accept defeat and to accept a lie but I continued to give in as if there was no way out.

A WAY OF ESCAPE
God always has an escape plan.

> **1 Corinthians:10:13,** *There hath no temptation taken you but such as is common to man: but God is faithful, who will not suffer you to be tempted above that ye are able; but will with the temptation also make a way to escape, that ye may be able to bear it.*

There were always ways of escape being made for me to take my exit, to take my next step in overcoming my stronghold, but I made the choice to remain in the suffering of my food addiction. I was not ready mentally to take the next step of being healed from it. It was comfortable, it was safe, and it was my place of solace. I knew that once I took the escape that exit that there was no returning back. The old Kia was going to be gone and I would have to embrace everything about the new Kia and let go of the old Kia and her ways.

The problem was I did not want to let go just so soon. I wanted to still enjoy my food and not feel any guilt, I wanted to continue on that path because at least then I was consistent with something. I did not want to leave only to return to the same unhealthy habits and feel like a failure.

I would attempt diets. I tried to be a vegetarian, I tried being a vegan, I tried the juice fast, I did the high protein diet, and meal replacements. I would stick to my diets, maybe lose 10 pounds or so and then fall back into the same unhealthy behavior patterns. Which would include eating out a lot, getting the appetizer, entree, and dessert and maybe even a cocktail. Almost every meal was prepared at a restaurant or some fast food place.

I would make attempts to exercise as well. I had a gym membership and would faithfully go until I got discouraged. I would not see results because I was still eating what I wanted to. By the way, I don't care what anybody says, you can't out exercise a bad diet! I even hired a personal trainer and that did not work for me either because, again, my eating habits were the same. This food thing was hard to conquer. It was really frustrating for me at times because I wanted to stop it but every time I tried, something would bring me back to the same patterns.

The Apostle Paul said in Romans 7:15, *"I do not understand what I do. For what I want to do I do not do, but what I hate, I do."*

This was my reality.

After a while, you can only kid yourself so much before the joke is on you. I don't know who I was trying to fool. I could lie to others and lie to myself, but I could not lie to God. He knew my wounds and how I really felt. I knew I wasn't living healthy, but I ignored God because I didn't want to admit I had a problem. My priorities were all messed up which lead to more unhealthy behavior patterns.

I love to dance so I would go out just so I could dance and have fun. I found since I gained weight and became more self-conscious I thought I needed to drink alcohol to take off the edge and numb the feeling of being uncomfortable in front of others. This was a vicious cycle. Alcohol is not only damaging to the liver but it is also full of empty calories and sugar and causes you to crave and eat unhealthy foods. In other words, it causes you to gain weight. So not only was I already overweight but I was trying to mask the fact that I was uncomfortable in my obesity by still going out and dressing nicely. All the while, I was drinking, which added to the weight gain.

Not only did it add to the weight gain but going out and dancing and consuming alcohol put me in vulnerable environments to be harassed even more. I was so lost that I did not even realize this. The problem I was running away from began to manifest because I was ignoring it.

I thought gone were the days of being sexually harassed now that I was an adult. I thought people knew how to keep their hands to themselves. A night on the town sure did prove me wrong. I vividly remember visiting one of my friends in Baltimore. We were out and about going to different bars and participating in the festivities. I was minding my own business enjoying the company of friends when this tall guy comes out of nowhere and slaps me on my butt.

My initial reaction was to hit, so I pushed him (this guy was like 6'4", but I didn't care). Then I said a few choice words to him. His defense was that he thought I was someone else. Even if that was the case, I don't care if it is a male friend or someone you are familiar with, no one has the right to violate your body or touch any parts of you unless you give them permission.

I was so embarrassed by this and very upset. The people I was hanging out with did not understand my frustration. They didn't know the depth of my wounds and how that incident brought up so many old issues and peeled back so many layers that I was not ready to reveal. I just wanted to leave and go home.

My night was ruined.

To make matters worse I continued to verbally get harassed by men as we were trying to get home.

The final straw came on a day I was teaching a Zumba class. From the class door of the studio, I noticed a "peeping Tom". Fortunately, one of my students witnessed this. She could see how uncomfortable I became and that I began to shut down. This prompted her to demand that he leave. I appreciated her standing up for me and coming to my rescue. I knew in order to defeat this issue I would have to stand up for myself. Between me witnessing her strength of being loud and vocal and of me being fed up, I said within myself enough is enough. I have put up with this for too long. I knew I had to stop being so spiritually timid. I got tired of feeling like a victim. I began to change my disposition from being afraid to being bold and fearless. Once I became more confident and bold in who I was, I noticed the harassment stopped. In hindsight, I realize this was a tactic of the enemy to keep me down, to rob me of my confidence, and rob me of the greatness that was inside of me.

I was one of those people that would pretend like I had it all together. Like nothing was wrong with me and

I was happy with being me. I put up a good facade and would justify my reasons of not wanting change.

I would say things to myself like, 'Men are still attracted to me so my body must not be so bad after all. I think I'll continue to stay the weight I am.'

I am wiser now and I know that relying on others for approval or acceptance only opens the door for rejection and disappointment because the same people you give power to place you on a pedestal can also use that same power you have given them to try to knock you down. I had to learn not to see my identity through human eyes, but through Christ.

THE GREAT PRETENDER

> ***Romans 12:2 (NIV)*** *says, 'Do not conform to the pattern of this world, but be transformed by the renewing of your mind. Then you will be able to test and approve what God's will is—His good, pleasing and perfect will.'*

My highest weight was 216 pounds. Deep down inside, I wanted out! I was tired of pretending. From the very beginning, I had to pretend that it didn't bother me that I couldn't swim in the pool with the other kids, I had to pretend like the lustful stares of men didn't bother me, and I had to pretend that I loved myself.

Yes. I said it. I had to pretend that I loved myself.

I had to pretend that when I put on a dress I liked the way it looked on my body. I had to pretend like I was ok with being in public and that it was comfortable.

By this point, I was so accustomed to being that size, and to my negative feelings about myself, that it just became second nature to think lowly of myself. I mean, I wanted to think highly of myself, I really did — but it is hard to look in the mirror and say you love what you see when you don't. It just made me more upset which made me want to eat more and more.

When you have reached the point where you are entangled in a lie and it's knotted so tightly, you lose your place of reference to where the lie starts and where it ends — you come to accept it as your truth. I surrendered to a lie for so many years that all of the spiritual, emotional, and mental weight I had been carrying for so many years was manifesting physically.

For the majority of my twenties, every time I went out, I wondered if people were judging me on my size. It kept me in anguish thinking of the perception people would have of me. It had gotten so bad that if I saw any old classmates from high school or college, I would try to avoid them. Taking the risk of anyone making a comment about my weight gain would have crushed what little iota of self-esteem I had left.

It was ironic that the same thing that brought me comfort, (food) was the very thing that caused my weight gain — which, in turn, brought me discomfort. The food and continuing weight gain had a tight grip on me and I was entangled in self-doubt and discouragement. There were things I wanted to do but didn't because my weight held me back. I became conscious of this cycle but could not figure how to escape its grasp.

Multiple attempts at dieting and exercise failed. I would lose weight but falter and end up quitting, no longer concerned about what I consumed or how much exercise I was getting. I was treating my body like it was trash, not like a temple. I was not treating it like a sacred place where my soul and Holy Spirit dwells. I was feeding it garbage. And as a result, I was producing garbage physically because of the extra burden of the ever-increasing weight I was placing on myself.

Because I was not taking care of my body physically, it begin to affect not only my body, but my mind and spirit as well. I would tell myself that I would be overweight for the rest of my life and would not be able to do the things I want to do anymore because there is no way I can lose weight. As a result of the lies I told myself, my spirit lacked confidence. My light had dimmed. There was no ambition and no desire to prosper and I was constantly low. It was so constant and I became so comfortable being in that posture that eventually I was contented with accepting defeat.

MODEL BEHAVIOR

I remember as a kid my aunts and I would watch fashion shows and admire supermodels such as Naomi Campbell or Cindy Crawford. In retrospect, I realize that just because they make it doesn't mean you have to buy it. Just because you see it in a magazine doesn't mean it is going to fit you the same way. The models in the fashion industry do not represent the average woman. They are beautiful in their own skin, however; we must realize that not everyone is tall and slim. Women come in different shapes, sizes, and heights.

As a child, I remember really wanting to be the size and height of those beautiful models. While I still love fashion shows and watching models strut their stuff on the runway, I am now able to appreciate it rather than get so caught up in wanting to be what I am not. As I became a mature adult, I realized that everyone cannot be that way and I had to learn to appreciate my body type and what clothes and styles work for me.

For example, I have big legs and I'm short so skirts that sit right above my knee make me look even shorter and my legs even bigger. I look better in either a skirt that is mid-thigh or that covers my knee, such as a pencil skirt. I used to think the bigger the clothes, the smaller I would look but proved to be quite the opposite. Bigger clothes made me look bigger as well. I used to want to wear long shirts to cover up my hips and tie jackets around my waist to cover up my butt, but that only made me look sloppy and heavier.

Finally, I realized, the more I try to hide my body the more I disgrace it — **so I began to embrace it.**

I discovered that clothes that accentuated my curves were complimentary to me. It took a while for me to be comfortable with wearing those types of clothes but I soon realized because I was not ashamed of my body, people were very receptive and would often compliment me on my clothes. I received so many compliments about the dress I wore to my high school prom one year.

There was one especially, given by a fellow classmate, that really made me feel good.

She said, "We were all talking about the dress you wore and how only you, with that body, could wear that dress."

It was then I realized that there is nothing wrong with being curvy and that we as women have the capability to empower one another.

I believe every woman has a style that works for her body type and it just takes a bit of trial and error to figure it out. We must understand that it is perfectly fine if the dress the runway model is wearing looks different on us and that just because it was made does not mean it was made for us. There are some dresses that look better on curvy women and some dresses that look better on slim women. It is up to us to figure out how can we can accentuate our best assets and be satisfied with that. When I shop for clothes, I don't adhere to what is considered popular or what everyone else is wearing. I go by what works for me and my body type, and what looks good on me — not the latest trend.

The thought of anyone touching me inappropriately without my permission just did something to me every time it would happen. It's as if it took away pieces of me. Every time I was violated I felt a loss of self and also feelings of anger and shame. Shame of my body and shame that it was drawing so much attention. I wanted to hide every piece of me. Over time I came to realize that it was not my fault if someone else could not control their behavior. A woman should not have to feel be ashamed of her assets even if it attracts unwanted attention.

Women can be hard on themselves and often feel the need to look in the mirror and pick apart every flaw. Women sometimes say put downs like "My butt is too big!" or "My boobs do not fit my body." Stop it! We must remove this negative thinking from our minds and realize we were created in God's image. So everything we see as a flaw, God's sees as perfection because we are His creation. And because of this, why then should we deny or reject what has already been established as beautiful? We were His idea when He formed the Earth.

Instead of taking ourselves apart with the negative thoughts we need to look in the mirror and say I love my God given (you fill in the blank).

I had to practice this myself. I had to look in the mirror and say I love my hips, they make me unique and they make the way I look in a dress unique. I love my butt and how it makes the way I look in jeans unique. I love my thighs, I love my big legs — I love my shape!!! I had to keep making myself look in the mirror even when there were times I did not want to. I had to force myself to like looking in the mirror and force myself appreciate my body. I had to accept the fact that I am short and curvy and I will never be a tall and slim runway model and I am just fine with that.

3

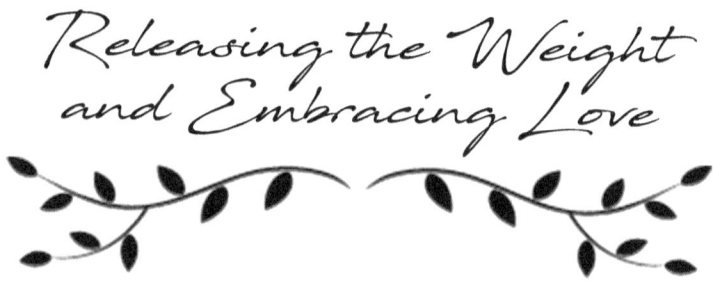
Releasing the Weight and Embracing Love

I remember the day so clearly. I was so embarrassed and didn't have a clue as to what I was going to do. I didn't know what I was going to say to my family or to my friends who had driven in from out of town just for this occasion.

So many thoughts raced through my mind like, 'God was this an answer to my prayers? Is this you working in the midst of what seems like one of the worse days of my life? What is going to come of this situation?'

I was so disconnected from Him; I couldn't recognize the signs earlier.

The month was October and I was preparing to celebrate my engagement with the person I thought I would marry at the time. Here I was on what was supposed to be one of the happiest days of my life.

It was supposed to be a celebration yet I was trying to find an excuse to why my fiancé at the time would not be able to show up. No one knew he was having a psychotic episode.

While all of my family was preparing and setting things up, I was trying to come up with reasons to cancel but I couldn't bring myself to do it. I was riddled with guilt because my dad had gone all out and spent a great deal of money on it. My uncle and aunt even opened up their beautiful home to host it in. I had to at least show up.

I was frantically hoping that my fiancé would pull through and that he would snap out of it. But, sadly, that's not how mental illness works. He was in no way capable of being in front of people in his state. He was delusional, paranoid, and manic. Even though he was not violent, it was still disturbing to be around him and people would definitely discern that something wasn't right. I wanted to protect him and his family did as well.

I could not face my family and friends with what was going on. Part of it was shame and part of it was pride. I had to have it all together and this messed up everything. I handled it the best way I knew how at the time by showing up without him...and I lied.

It was not my proudest hour. For some of my family and friends reading this, this will be the very first time discovering the truth. How was I going to say that he couldn't show up because he's going crazy? Instead, I told them he was admitted to the emergency room and I have since repented and asked for forgiveness for deceiving them. In my mind, I lied to cover him and cover my humiliation.

How could I not see the signs? How could I not see the person I was with for 4 years was suffering from a mental illness? How could I not recognize this? Had I been so completely blind and oblivious or was I just that desperate to get married? Could it be I stuck it out so long, even though it wasn't the healthiest situation, just so in the end it would result in a ring and a marriage? How did I miss the mark? So I did what I knew how to do best. I covered up, pretended, put on a smile, socialized, and laughed. I acted as though I was not breaking down inside. As if inside, I was not experiencing my own chaotic world of confusion — of questions — of vulnerability. I stayed as long as I could and then I left the party to go back to the house of someone who was being tormented mentally, who was delusional, depressed, and irrational. I went from being a significant other to a care taker. That day began one of the worst seasons of my life.

I was too ashamed to tell anyone the truth just yet. Mental illness is a taboo in most societies and I myself did not have the language to explain what was happening. Too often, people joke or use mental disorders loosely to describe someone they deem as not normal and I certainly did not want to face the judgement of other people. I did not think they would understand and I felt very lonely.

How do I even begin to explain the details?

The discouragement further abounded with my attempt to confide in a friend who had experienced something similar with her husband. I was pouring out my heart and telling her all that I was going through but her response was not quite what I expected. The lack of compassion and apathy I was hearing on the other end on the phone was enough to for me to know who I could really depend on when times were tough and it was not her. This was surprising to me as I had been there for her through some of her darkest and most embarrassing moments. She made me feel as though I was inconveniencing her with my phone call and she did not have the time to listen.

As I began to reflect on how I was treated, nothing about our friendship was convenient for me, yet I valued her as a person and understood the tough times she was going through. I did not want to add salt to a wound so I never complained about it.

That phone call was the last time we spoke. I was expecting her to at least check on me with a text or email if she did not have the time to talk. However, my expectations were too high. It did not take long for me to realize that this friendship had reached its final destination. This was something I had to let go of and be at peace about it. I waited months before finally sending her a text stating that the last couple of months had been really tough for me and it would have been nice to have heard from her. Needless to say, there was no reply but I did not send the text for a reply I sent it for closure on my part. I was releasing the weight of anyone who added debt to my life.

In that experience, I learned the priceless lesson on how to give the gift of goodbye — of how to let go of people, places, and things that added no value to my life. In that season of releasing the weight, if the relationships I had with people did not add up, I would ask myself "what am I fighting for?" If my answer did not make sense, I had to release them from my life.

Releasing people from your life that add no value to it is not a bad thing, it does not mean you are a bad person. However, it does send a message that you are loyal to your happiness & wellbeing. Guess what?!? **Spoiler Alert!** There is nothing wrong with being loyal to the standards and values you set for your life. There is nothing wrong with concluding that if people cannot recognize your worth, you can make it easier on them by removing yourself from their life. It is just that simple. There does not have to be a dramatic scene or a big argument. What I have learned is there are a lot of people on this Earth and God will bless you with more friends, more confidants, and more relationships. There is always a blessing on the other side of detoxing from people who are not good for your life.

THE COLORS OF THE SEASON

If I could paint a picture of that season it would include prisms of reds, oranges, blues, greens, and browns. It was autumn and the air was crisp with notes of cool breezes and warm kisses from the sun. The skies were a soft baby blue with variations of white clouds in each of their respective places. The grass was covered with the beautiful adornment of fall leaves. The colors would also symbolize the internal picture I had on the inside. The red would symbolize my brokenness and the bleeding of wounds. The blues would symbolize that depressed state I begin to experience and the coldness of the season as winter approached. The season where your bones begin to ache from the chill of a frost, where you begin to see your breath dissipate in the air with every word spoken. The season where you begin to cover up more to keep warm, to protect yourself from the chilling cold air. This season was symbolic of what I was going through. I begin to cover up my emotions and feelings with layers of pride, a layer of "strong independent woman." Not realizing I was not in control all along.

There is always an event that stops you in your tracks and lets you know that you are not in charge. For me, that event was the death of my dear younger brother.

It was a Christmas morning I will never forget. My dad called early that morning. I knew something must have been wrong because he usually does not call me that early. Then he uttered the words I would never forget…"Javon died." I said, "What?" because clearly I was half asleep and didn't hear him correctly. Clearly it was a nightmare I was having or a bad joke. I know my brother, he could not have died — he could not be gone. He loved life and he was sweet. I just saw him on Thanksgiving.

He repeated himself. I became distraught and could not believe the news I was receiving, and of all the days, on Christmas morning. I thought my life was over. First my fiancé is suffering from a mental illness and now my brother is dead. I couldn't believe it. Was I being punished? I couldn't understand how so many things could go wrong at once. How was I supposed to deal with all of this? Life began to get real and it became too much for me. Life hit me so hard that the impact could be compared to that of a tractor trailer going 100 miles per hour right into a brick wall. My world was completely turned around. It hit me so hard that it paralyzed me. The events paralyzed my thoughts and my being. Little did I know, that the worse season of my life, was setting me up for destiny.

In the midst of my season of grief and loss, I did not recognize God's glory. He was answering my prayers by showing me signs of why the person I was considering for marriage was not a good candidate. My fiancé at the time, during his psychotic episodes, would share (confess) with me about all the times he cheated on me and that he was sorry for it. Every hidden and dark thing came to surface. On top of losing my brother, I was losing someone I cared for and thought I was going to spend the rest of my life with as well. It was during this time that I learned that God answers prayers — even if the answer is presented in a way that we don't expect. I had enough information to make an informed decision to end that relationship. When I knew I could not rely on my own strength, it was time I went back to the Source.

ESTRANGED FATHER

Before all of these tragedies occurred, I was the furthest away from God that I could have ever been. Our relationship was estranged yet He never stopped loving me. Somewhere the signals got mixed up and I begin to do my "own thing."

Sure there were times where I prayed, sure there were times where I read the Bible, sure there were times I visited churches, but I thought, 'What's the use? I have no value to offer.' I literally thought that God did not love me. That because I did not pursue a relationship with Him, He had stopped pursuing a relationship with me — but that was never the case. I now understand God doesn't work that way. His thoughts are higher than our thoughts and His ways are higher than our ways.

I took two weeks of bereavement leave and it was the first in a while, that I was <u>still.</u> The Bible tells us to 'be still and know that I am God'. At the time, I didn't have much Word in me then so I didn't know that scripture. But that is why it's called the 'living word' because it was (and still is) active in my life at a time that I needed it the most. I was living out the passage by just sitting and being still and quiet. I had to get in the face of God and surrender. My spirit knew what to do and it yearned for more of the Father.

In those two weeks, I began to journal and reflect on my life. I wondered what happened to me. What happened to that ambition I had? What happened to those dreams I had? How did I become so unhealthy?

God began to deal with me and reminded me that after all these years He had never left me. He never forgot about me. He brought back to my memory events from my past and issues that I had buried so deep I had literally erased them from my memory. There were issues I misplaced and feelings I covered up. He brought everything to the surface and I could no longer hide from my past. Those two weeks were the beginning of my journey to pursuing destiny.

You see, sometimes it takes a tragedy happening or for life to really disrupt some things for you to understand your purpose; for you to begin to question, for you to begin to explore, for you to begin to start your transformation. You have to know that in order to get better, in order to prosper or really be who God has designed you to be, there is going to have to be a moment of truth — a moment of reflection, a moment where you begin to realize that there are some mistakes you made and there are some things you missed that contributed to your own detour or your own delay.

I know firsthand how faithful God is. I know that no matter how far you go astray, God will still tug on you and lead you into the direction you need to go. It was in that time that even though it did not feel the best — even though I was hurting and I was breaking down, my life as I knew was crumbling before me, and everything was turned upside down — it was in those times he was preparing me. He was setting me up to walk into my destined place.

In retrospect, if it had not been for the disappointments, the heartbreak, the grief and the pain, I would not be the person I have become today. That was my season of pruning, that was my season of shedding and that was my season of *releasing the weight.*

RELEASING THE WEIGHT

I know most people are familiar with the term "losing weight" but I purposely chose *releasing the weight* to describe my transformation process. You see, to lose something means it happened by accident or by mistake but when you *release* something you are making an *intentional* decision to let go. For example, if I lose my car keys and someone finds them and takes my car; that is an accidental loss that I made no preparation for. But if I release my car keys to someone else for them to drive it, I am making an intentional decision to let them go.

As I made the intentional decision to let go of some people, forgive past hurts, and face my fears head on; I began to not only see a change spiritually, mentally, and emotionally — but physically. My appetite for food changed. I no longer needed the satisfaction of food to fill a void in my life. I no longer craved the comfort of a meal but I was in search of something more, something meaningful.

Relationships, emotional eating, and other bad habits were all void fillers to what I was really missing in my life — my relationship with Jesus Christ. In seeking Him, I was able to bring to surface every hidden and dark area of my life. He allowed me to work on me and covered me in the process. As I was releasing the weight I became empowered and fragile all at the same time.

There was one scripture I remember my Big Mama (grandmother) telling me and I committed to memorize that scripture. It was Isaiah 40:31. It said, *But they that wait upon The Lord shall renew their strength; they shall mount up with wings as eagles; they shall run, and not be weary; and they shall walk, and not faint.* At the time I did not have much of God's Word in me but reciting that passage empowered me. Even to this day, I get fired up reading it.

If you are enduring a hard season in your life and you do not know the Bible thoroughly, you can start anywhere and memorize something — even if that is the only scripture you can hold to memory. That is one more scripture you did not know and one more scripture that is building you and strengthening your faith. Don't compare yourself to those who are gifted at commanding the word. *Your journey is your journey.* If you are faithful over learning a few, God will supernaturally increase your ability to retain more of His Word and revelation. I am a living witness — I went from barely knowing any scriptures to being a licensed and ordained preacher of the Gospel.

Because of everything I was going through, it became difficult to function at work or during my daily activities. I was becoming more and more depressed by the sudden and abrupt changes in my life and did not even realize it was happening. My depression, sprinkled with grief and mourning, caused me to start a cycle of sleeping more than I was living. I would literally get off work and stay in the bed from 6 p.m. until 7 a.m. the next morning. There was no desire to be social or hangout with friends. I would screen my calls and the majority of the time my voicemail box would be full as that seemed like the best location for the calls I did not want to take. I shut people out and in the process I was shutting down.

    Releasing mental, emotional, physical, and spiritual weight is a process. I was going through a holistic detox. I was getting rid of toxic things in my life that hindered my growth. Anytime you begin to detox, the experience is not always pleasant. Things seem to actually feel worse before they get better. I felt every bit of the side effects of detoxing. I felt withdrawal, I felt pain, I felt deprived, and I felt the sacrifice.

    I say sacrifice because that is what it felt like as I let go of things I had held on to for so long. I knew I needed some help with that process. I wanted to get back to my old self again — I wanted to be able to function and I wanted to enjoy life again. I could see myself going further and further into a downward spiral. But then, one day, I came to myself and I said, 'ENOUGH'!

    One of the benefits my job offered was the Employee Assistance Program (EAP) and I took advantage of it. It gave me the much needed opportunity to talk to a mental health professional. It was so important for me to be able to talk to someone that wasn't biased, who would listen, and was a professional. It's funny because my intentions were to only go to get advice on how to cope with my mentally unhealthy fiancé at the time. However, God had another plan. He led me to the right person and to that place for a reason. What was supposed to be three sessions, ended up being a weekly appointment for about a year.

I felt comfortable enough to share my deepest hurt and get everything that had happened to me off of my chest. At the time, I had only shared with very few people the details of my life (I was too embarrassed to tell them the whole story). The therapy sessions really allowed me to purge and work on expressing my feelings in a healthy way and not feel as though I had to hide them.

I believe God is the ultimate Healer and Source and He uses resources or vessels to help along the way. Everybody has a different process, and for me, therapy was a part of mine. It was my safe place because it was hard for me to be honest with myself. The sessions also allowed me to further explore my childhood and understand the root cause of the issues I had that were holding me back.

REMOVING DISTRACTIONS

Distractions allow us to lose focus of our purpose, of our proper alignment, and of our passion. There were many distractions going on in my life that contributed to my internal battles with myself. Those distractions included engaging in the wrong activities and clinging to dysfunctional relationships.

I used to be an avid television watcher. I was addicted to reality TV, watching music videos, and whatever the latest greatest show was. As long as it brought me entertainment and as long as I could escape reality and get engulfed in it, I was content with sitting on the couch being idle.

Idleness is the devil's workshop. If you are not being productive it will cause you to rot spiritually, physically, mentally and emotionally. Spiritually, I was not being fed. I was malnourished with the garbage that I was watching on television. My guidance became what the world thought and how the world acted.

When you are sitting down all the time and not moving your muscles they begin a process called atrophy or to deplete in mass. Muscles are essential in burning calories while at rest. They are essential for movement and for strength. The weaker your muscles are the more out of shape you can become causing fatigue in many daily activities such as lifting groceries. The heart is a muscle and a vital organ. Exercise and movement helps keep the heart in good condition. Finally, the more TV you watch the more emotionally attached you are to it.

We all have a favorite TV show we like or must see every week. Why? Because we are emotionally invested. The shows we watch either make us laugh, cry, excited, angry or confused. Either way, it stimulates us. Thus, watching too much of it can cause us to be over stimulated and if we are not careful, these emotions can be overwhelming — which can trigger other issues such as overeating. It also doesn't help that the commercials on television advertise enticing food and restaurant deals that make you feel like you just have to have it. I can remember there was a time where I would be full and finished with my last meal of the day. Then I would see a commercial about some new dessert or some new dish and I would all of a sudden become hungry. Well, that wasn't hunger; that was greed. I wanted more and more because I knew it would make me feel good and it would make me happy. Especially if it was as good as the advertisement said it would be.

Watching television all day can cause depression or stress which is not a good thing when it comes to mental health. Once something gets implanted in your mind it can overtake your whole being. Then, before you know it you are trapped wondering how did I get here? How is it that I am eating so much and never full or satisfied? Why do I feel overwhelmed with emotions all the time? Why can't I get to the gym and exercise? Why aren't I motivated? It's because you have gotten too comfortable and complacent.

Because I was not content with me and I did not fully love myself, I was constantly seeking approval from others. I thought if someone loved me enough it would possibly help me love myself more as well. If someone appreciates my body in a healthy way that makes me feel comfortable then maybe I can appreciate my body more. This was a twisted way of thinking and if you are someone that feels this way please get to a place where your approval does not lie in other people. It is called codependence and is unhealthy in many ways. Pray for strength to not depend on man's approval and receive God's approval (Romans 3:24) and what he says about you. That is where you will find truth about yourself not in what man says.

When you give the wrong people too much power they can abuse the responsibility you have allowed them to have and it can hurt you more than help you. When someone feels like they have authority over you and they don't know how to handle it properly, it can lead to abuse. Verbal abuse can cause damage even if you don't accept what that person is telling you. If you are constantly hearing it, it causes you to eventually believe it. This type of behavior can be demonstrated among family members, significant others, or people you may think are your friends. What God says about you never changes but what man says about you can, depending on what mood they are in.

If a family member was miserable and wanted someone to pick on, I would be first choice because they knew that my weight and self-image was a wound for me. So I would be attacked in that area by unpleasant words such as, "that's why you're fat!" That is why it is so important to know who you are and where your identity lies. People are fickle minded and have their own issues but God is not a man that he should lie and his Word always stands true.

For a while my self-esteem was destroyed because of the lies I had been told by people I trusted. Once I removed those distracting relationships out of my life, I was able to prosper, focus and heal. It took me years because removing people who are family out of your life is not an easy task. However there comes a time where you learn how to love from a distance. You keep them in prayer and you can be there for them in times of need, but **you have to set boundaries and let go.** Otherwise it will be difficult to have a healthy idea of yourself.

    If you really want to know how to love yourself you must first accept God's love. I remember a time in my life where it was hard for me to accept God's love and blessings. Whenever something good happened to me, I would feel guilt and anxiety. All I could think was something bad was just around the corner waiting to happen. When my brother died and I went through that season of grief and loss, God taught me how to be loved. He used the most unlikely people to show me love and through the people I thought would be there for me but weren't, He showed me what love was not. At my most vulnerable moment and during one of the toughest times of my life, God showed me who to leave behind and who to keep. Although it hurt me, I had no choice but to disconnect from those who were apathetic towards me in my time of grief.

    I slowly but surely began to accept and receive God's love. When all of my co-workers attended my brother's funeral and were there to support me — that was God's love. When my co-worker saw I was having a hard time and gave me some advice — that was God's love. When my other co-worker gifted me a day at the spa to help relieve some of the stress I was experiencing — that was God's love. When my college friends reached out every now and then to come visit me and hangout— that was God's love. When my best friends sent me a care package to cheer me up — that was God's love. I was just overwhelmed by all of the support and all of God's favor upon me. His love covers a multitude of sin and His love was healing for me in my time where I felt the most vulnerable and alone.

If you want to be taught how to love look at God's love for us:
1. *He will never leave or forsake us*
2. *He doesn't hold grudges*
3. *He is selfless*
4. *He is a comforter*
5. *He is a liberator*

The problem was not *if* He loved me or *how much* He loved me — because I know his love is unconditional — the real issue was that I had to realize His love. I did not realize where I stood with God. I thought God only loved the people who diligently served Him who were "good" Christians and never made mistakes. Well, we know there is no such thing as someone who does not make mistakes. But yet I still thought He only paid special attention to the leaders in the church or to those with titles. I was insecure in my relationship with God which affected my faith and affected my identity — and because of my identity crisis I was not able to fully receive the love of God or grasp the concept of agape love. Often times we look at what God is doing for other people and feel left out or like we are not worthy of the same blessings but God has no respect of persons. He is omnipresent and His love is endless.

If you're not comfortable with yourself or if you don't love yourself completely, I would suggest you not entertain the idea of being in a relationship. **No person can fill that void.** Your insecurities will give that person too much power — the power to build you up or tear you down. This is very dangerous. It is unhealthy because you're depending on another human being to dictate how you feel. You have to look to God for your strength and what he says about you. It is in his Word that you find peace and understanding not in the words of man.

I used to be all too guilty of this. My first boyfriend, my high school sweetheart whom I depended on to make me feel like my body was ok, had to endure my bouts of negative body image moments. That must have been frustrating and exhausting for him. I would constantly ask does this make me look fat, does my butt look big in this? He would constantly tell me, "You're perfect, you're beautiful, I love you just the way you are. Please don't change a thing". He would always say that I was beautiful but even that was not enough because I did not believe it myself so I could not trust someone else's word. **I wish, back then, I had enough of God's Word in me to know my true identity.** Perhaps I would not have had meltdowns every time I tried on something that didn't fit right or made me look "big."

That same boyfriend invited me over his house to spend Christmas with him and his family and on that Christmas he gifted me some knee length boots. I was so excited because I had always wanted a pair! But I wasn't prepared for what happened next — I tried them on and couldn't get them past my calf. I was devastated and out of frustration I began to cry. I felt embarrassed because this was a Christmas present that was supposed to bring me joy and it did the opposite. It was like, once again my body failed me; and if I had skinny legs, I would not have this problem. I wanted so badly to wear them. I should have realized that it wasn't the fact that my legs were too big but the design of the boot was not made for females with big calves. The extended calf idea did not come into existence until later and I am so glad that designers finally came to the realization that every woman is not the same.

Instead of me having a breakdown and completely feeling like my world was crashing down, I could have had a different perspective or mindset on things. Instead I let something that was man-made — something that was temporary and could be destroyed — control how I felt about myself. How crazy is that?

My mindset was all wrong. To change the way you view your body you have to rearrange your mind set. Not make excuses, but rearrange. There is a difference. Excuses cover up, like putting a band-aid on it; they dress it up but don't really fix the issue. That allows you to remain comfortable and does not promote healing. Figuring out the cause of the wound is what causes restoration. Rearranging your mind allows you to view things in a different perspective and in a different light. It changes your thoughts and outlook. If I had the mindset that I had today, my journey would have been that much easier. I would have been confident in myself and would not have had to rely on others to determine if my look was acceptable. I would have been more accepting to my flaws and to my body. I would have not looked from within to point the blame.

Loving yourself is necessary because it is a commandment from God. The Bible says love God first then your neighbor as you love yourself (Matthew 22:39). So therefore if you don't love yourself, you can't possibly be able to love your neighbor. If we want to please God we must be obedient to his commandments and love Him then love ourselves as we love others.

4

The Launching

Rockets are used by NASA to launch people or things into space. They work from the principle of Newton's Third Law of Motion; for every action there is an equal and opposite reaction. The same massive force (action) that is generated by hot gases firing backward from a rocket's engines produces an equal force (reaction) that pushes the rocket forward through space.

The same concept can be applied to our lives; as the same force or burden of the vision you are carrying gets stronger, the equal reaction causes you to push forward and give birth to your destiny. God was my rocket! He took all the heat and fuel (action) from my past to cause a launching (reaction) into my future.

In therapy, I learned so much about myself; how much I compromised myself for so long, how much I would hide my truth, and how I did more thinking than feeling. I also learned that as I was beginning to work on improving my mental and emotional state; taking care of my physical, as well as spiritual health was just as important. I began to believe in myself again. The dreams that were buried and those things I wanted to do before, suddenly became possible to achieve. I was beginning to feel like I had a purpose on this Earth that God wanted to use me to help others who may have struggled with their body image or weight or self-esteem.

One of the things I knew God was calling me to do was become a health and wellness coach and help people in that area. Through my own experience of releasing the weight, I knew first hand that exercise and eating right was not enough when it came to being a healthy person. If your spirit is filled with godliness, it affects your thoughts, it affects your feelings and it affects your temple.

With this charge in my spirit, I stepped out on faith and the process of branding myself as a health and wellness coach was underway. The credentials were already in place. I had a Bachelor of Science in Community Health Education and a Master's in Public Health which meant, not only did I have the knowledge, but I also possessed the real life experience necessary to start my business. I was embarking on new territory of entrepreneurship and filled with so many mixed emotions. I was excited, nervous, and scared all at once.

It was about a ten month process from the time I began to see myself as a health and wellness coach to the time of the actual launching of my business. First, there was some ground work that needed to be done. I had to take everything that was in my head and translate it into a concrete business plan. There were also some tangible things I needed to have in place such as a website, content for my website (blog posts, my services, and biography), business cards, a logo, social media graphics; and, to top it all off, I needed to be coached in being a savvy business woman.

Even though I knew this was a God-idea, I still had that strong hold of doubt and insecurity trying to talk me out of pursuing purpose. I would have moments of feeling on top of the world to moments where thoughts like, 'who is going to believe I'm a health coach', plagued my mind. To be honest, I was not completely delivered from lacking confidence in myself and did not realize at the time that I gave myself too much credit. I did not see that the process would have been a lot smoother if I just placed more of my confidence in Jesus rather than in my own abilities. I knew God wanted me to do this so it was imperative that I not give up — no matter how uncomfortable it was for me. I had sacrificed so much and invested way too much money to just walk away. I knew I had to try!

I believed so much in the vision God gave me, that I would sometimes not pay a bill in order to fund my efforts. At times, I would go without groceries and meals just to make sure I had everything I needed in place. It was during this season that my faith and trust in God increased. He truly showed me that He was my provider. There were times when I did not have lunch and someone at work would offer to take me to lunch. There were times that I was on my last dime and did not know how I was going to pay for gas or food before the next pay check but somehow I would run into money. There were times where I went to church with my gas tank nearly on E and I would leave church with enough money for gas and food. I am not revealing this to brag or boast and I do not recommend anyone do what I did unless they are clearly hearing the voice of God leading them in that direction. I understood in that season it was necessary for me to endure those things in order to have a closer relationship to Him and to grow spiritually.

FINISH STRONG

Despite the financial challenges I ran into during the beginning stages of my business, I was determined to finish what I started. I had set a date to officially launch my website and could not think of a better date than my birthday. What better day to give birth to a divine vision than the day God decided to place me on the Earth? I was so excited! I could not wait. Finally, my dreams were coming true and after going through hell and back the previous year, people would see God's glory. If He was able to use me despite my circumstances and all I had been through, then He could use anybody. For so long I did not believe in myself and that I could even pursue teaching people how to live healthier lives because I was so unhealthy myself. I was finally going to be able to share with the world the purpose behind all that I had been through.

The time was 11:59 p.m. I was only moments away from officially sharing with everyone on social media what God was doing in my life. It was a surreal moment. In a matter of seconds the website would be seen by all my social media friends and family. I knew once I hit the send button there was no turning back. This was my new truth. I had a date with destiny and I was going to show up. From that point on my life would forever change. My perspective changed and I was walking in a newness of life.

That night, I debuted my website — iamkiapotts.com — and got such positive feedback. People were congratulating me and messaging me with encouraging words. It was all the more confirmation to let me know that every tear and sacrifice was worth it. Some people would message me telling me how one of my blog posts helped them get through a difficult time or break-up. It was mind blowing and I could not believe God was using me in that way.

Later, I got the idea to have an official website launch party at the place where I taught my Zumba classes called: *A New You Wellness Center*. I thought it would be a great way to bring people together to promote health and wellness as well as promote the website. This would be a huge undertaking for me because it would mean taking on the dual role of party planner and host. By the grace of God, I was able to get the majority of the event sponsored. The owner of *A New You Wellness Center* donated the venue, my church paid for the door prizes, my daddy paid for the catering, and my mom helped me set up. However, In the middle of planning the launch party, I began to get discouraged.

Where I was once feeling triumphant, self-doubt and anxiety were rearing their ugly heads again. There was even a period I stopped promoting the website launch event out of fear that either no one would support it or I would not have everything I needed to have a successful event. I was on the brink of canceling it until one day my pastor noticed a change in my enthusiasm. He asked how the planning process was coming along and I began to tell him how I was no longer excited about it. I had allowed my fears and worries to choke out my momentum and victory. Encouraging me, he said that I had to do this because it was needed in the community. His affirming message to me was just what I needed to hear to get back to business as usual. After that, I started to heavily promote the event and the RSVP's were rolling in.

The event was a success and symbolized a pivotal moment in my life. Yes it was a launch party for my website, but it was also the start to God launching me into my destiny. I was created to do this. I was created to do the type of work that inspires people to live healthier so that they may prosper in all areas of life and always give God the glory. There was such an outpouring of support at the website launch party from family, friends, people that participated in my Zumba classes, and strangers. I gave away prizes to the winners of the fitness contests I had. There were jump rope, sit-up, plank, and hula hoop contests. The entire night was filled with good clean fun and healthy eats.

There is something so fulfilling about seeing a vision come to fruition. God gives us these creative downloads and insights to our future, and once we see His promises come to pass, there's a feeling of pure gratification knowing that the Father is pleased. That was the feeling I felt that night after the launch party. I felt as though I could conquer anything. After sacrificing so much to start this health coaching business and after almost giving up on having a launch party, I now understood that the reward for being faithful is far greater than the comfort of giving up.

DIETARY CHANGES

For so many years I tried to just focus on physically losing weight and would be so unsuccessful. Now I was going to get the opportunity to help others who may have been in a cycle of unsuccessful attempts at achieving their health and wellness goals. I did not realize that the reason why I was making the wrong choices in natural foods was because it was a reflection of the choices I was feeding my mind, emotions, and spirit.

I served my mind large portions of junk which included but was not limited to: doubt, negative thinking, and lies. I spent too much time in front of the television watching meaningless shows and not enough time in the Word of God or in prayer. The Bible tells us that bodily exercise profits little but exercise yourself in godliness for it profits in all things, this life and eternity. This is so true because once I found a church home where I could exercise my godliness and grow in Christ, my health prospered tremendously.

My priorities shifted. I made more time and effort to attend services such as Bible Study and Midnight Prayer that would strengthen and feed my mind and spirit. I was intentional about my transformation to grow spiritually. Every time the church doors were opened, I was there. I sacrificed weekend trips to visit my friends in D.C. because I knew it was important to be in attendance on Sunday mornings and I did not want to risk missing out on anything. More importantly, I was seeing the results of my sacrifice paying off. I was so happy and content. Sunday became my favorite day of the week. I looked forward to spending time with my church family. I looked forward to hearing my pastor preach an inspiring, thought provoking and substantial message. Once I purposely made changes to live more holy, I realized that I did not want to go back to my previous lifestyle.

I was at peace and it felt like nothing was missing. Sure I had my moments of challenges and trials; but overall, in that season of rededicating my life back to Christ, I realized the feeling that I felt was what I had been looking for my entire life — and that was *wholeness*.

5

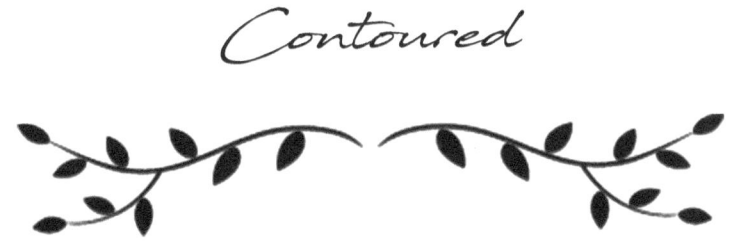

Contoured

con·tour: ˈkän ˌto͝or/verb past tense: contoured; past participle: contoured.

To mold into a specific shape, typically one designed to fit into something else.

The definition of contoured is to mold into a specific shape, typically one designed to fit into something else. I did not realize it at the time, but day by day I was being molded into someone else to please another person and fit into their standard of beauty and quality when in reality there was nothing wrong with me. What I could not understand is that the same person that once called me beautiful without make-up was now complaining that I did not have enough of it on. How did I get to a place where I allowed someone to make me feel as though

80 Naked and Not Ashamed

I was not good enough? How did this happen — to me of all people? I was free; I was confident and beautiful. How did I let this go so far? The reality is this can happen to any woman and that is why it is so important to be ok with someone walking away from your life even if it means you will be alone for a season. I was so focused on fulfilling a dream of being married and having kids that I was willing to try to fit into someone else's image for me and not God's image of me.

It was all very calculating. He was looking for a wife — but not just any wife; he was looking for a First Lady. That's right, he was a pastor. I remember the first message I received from him. I couldn't believe he was inboxing me, let alone, communicating with me at all. He barely spoke two words to me when I would see him in person and now he is talking to me? Initially, I think I was so stuck on the fact that a pastor was interested in me that there were some red flags I either ignored, justified, or was in denial about.

There are multiple pivotal moments in our lives. There are those moments when we learn the other side of love and experience our first heartbreak, there are moments where we experience so much joy it's almost like an utopian feeling, there are moments we may experience great grief or tragedy, there are moments where everything under the sun is funny, and then there are moments where we are content just being. When we know that life has more to offer us but we are ok with waiting and we don't allow future promises to diminish our present.

I remember being this way when I first joined my church. I had gone through so much in previous years that when I finally found a church home, I finally had some idea of who I was in Christ and I was finally implementing all the visions and dreams I had buried after experiencing one disappointment after another. My soul was resting and I was fine being me. Metaphorically speaking, I was fine being in the garden naked and not ashamed. Like the garden experience, I was faced with choices. I made the choice to see where the journey would take me in hopes that eventually marriage would be the destination. Sometimes in life you make choices and then there are times where choices make you. This choice "made me", alright. It made me think twice about responding to Facebook inbox messages. It made me more cautious. It made me see that people are people and titles do not exempt you from being human. It also made me not be so quick to assume people should act or be a certain way because they are in ministry.

It was a lovely Sunday afternoon. I had just finished having a fun time at my church's Father's Day cookout and I was preparing to leave for my vacation in Florida the next day. I remember the first friend request I received from him. I didn't think anything of it.

Then I received the typical "Thanks for accepting my friend request" message.

"You're welcome" I replied.

A day or two would pass and he would try to make small talk about something. I still didn't think much of it. It was not until he began to ask questions like: "Age,"

"Do you have children," "How long have you been saved," that I realized he was interested in me. Within the first week of exchanging phone numbers we talked multiple times during the day and sometimes Facetimed each other. I was so excited about this. I thought, "Wow, God! You must be rewarding me for honoring you in my singleness and being faithful to You." Little did I know, my self-esteem and value and everything I worked so hard to overcome, would soon be tested.

At the time, I didn't know what I was more excited about; that God's promise to me was going to be fulfilled, that I had met the "one"; or the fact that he was a pastor. That alone made me feel special. A pastor wants me? I never thought of myself as being a "Pastor's Wife" or a wife of any man that was very distinguished and godly. I thought only women from prestigious backgrounds or who have been in church all of their lives marry men like that. His approaching me definitely boosted my self-esteem. I thought, "Wow. I must be doing something right for him to notice me. Out of all the women he could have because of his position, he's interested in me." I couldn't believe it.

In hindsight, this was a clear indicator that I had no business being in any relationship. Unbeknownst to me, there were still some parts of me that needed healing and that I needed to be whole in.

Why couldn't I see myself as a pastor's wife or a woman of prestige? Still in the developing stage, I had not fully received a revelation of how God saw me, so I trusted a man's view of me. God was still perfecting me.

There are four steps to *perfection*. Perfection, meaning, being whole or complete in Christ. There is **the kneading, the molding, the drying, and the firing.** Yes, the same process in which a potter molds a piece of clay is the same process in which God begins to work on us.

The kneading is when God begins to remove the debris and impurities from us.

The molding is when God places His hands on us and begins to shape us into the image in which He wants us to be. He begins to show us who we are and our purpose and our use in the Earth.

The drying is the season in which we have to sometimes sit and be still because we are fragile at this point. We are not fully ready to go forth; it's our preparation season.

The final stage is **the firing**. It's so important that we are ready for the firing because if we are not, we will get easily discouraged in pursuing destiny. Once you enter into the firing you are making a covenant with The Potter that you will not be moved by life's circumstances or the opinions of others. You are making a permanent decision because the pottery becomes nearly indestructible once it goes through the fire.

The issue was I allowed him to be my potter and not God. That is, he began to mold me and shape me into his ideal of me. I started to become the expectation he wanted instead of being what God designed and the disappointing part is that I allowed it. I didn't realize that while he was sending me videos on how to contour my face (a makeup technique), he was trying to get me to contour my life as well. I was being molded into a box, his box; which was filled with impossible ideologies and concepts that were ridiculous and superficial all to feel accepted by a pastor with hopes of one day being his wife.

When we first started talking on the phone, I was excited I could actually talk about God with a man, and he was even more excited to talk about God with me. This was exactly what I wanted; a man that could share insight and revelation with me, pray with and for me, speak into my life, and to add to the conversation, he valued my views and my relationship with Christ. I thought for once in my life, I actually have a relationship that is Christ-centered. Even more, I felt special because not only did we have long discussions on how awesome God is but he already made me feel as though I was his wife.

He would make statements such as '*when* (not if) we get married' and '*when* we have kids'. Those were very declarative statements. He would rehearse his sermons with me, ask me to pray for him before his preaching engagements, and confide in me about his plans and visions for the church he pastored. He would even tell me about issues and things that happened from time to time at his church. All of this made me feel important and like I belonged, and that was enough for me to trust him. So when he made a suggestion about me getting my clothes tailor-made at his expense, I allowed it. It was not obvious to me at the time that his suggestions really meant he was unhappy with my looks. I took it as if he just wanted to do something nice for me because he liked me so much.

One of my love languages is receiving gifts. Therefore, I did not think much of it when he bought me shoes, coats, dresses, purses and jewelry. Then one day, out of nowhere, he made a comment I would never forget.

"No one has ever said anything to you about your looks?" he said.

At this point, I was offended and said, "No. No one has ever complained until now."

He continued to say, "You have all the qualities I want in a wife, I just do not like the way you dress."

By this time, I was upset. He went on to say that he would get anxiety about going on a date with me because he had no idea what I would wear — as if I was going to embarrass him. I was completely crushed. This should have been my cue to exit but by this time I was already six months into the relationship which in my mind meant I was closer to being engaged and married. Again, I was still holding on to the dream of having it all. Sadly, I put up with it because I thought that it was something I could adjust to please him. But soon he began to critique more than my clothes.

I would take pictures of my outfit just for his approval which started to get very unhealthy for my self-esteem. If he approved, I felt great; if he disliked anything, I felt awful. How did I end up back in the place of being dependent on another person's opinion to validate me? Eventually, I began to depend on his approval far too often and felt like I was walking on eggshells around him. When it came to being around him, my freedom was limited because he was so critical of everything. So I would just shut down. It was hard to be myself in an environment like that. I knew I had to let go but I just did not know how.

"God help me to see me the way You see me," I would pray, so that I could build my esteem back up and depend on God's affirmations for approval.

One minute he would be nice and say the sweetest things, another minute he would have some type of negative or disapproving remark. The lesson that I learned while in the midst of that ordeal was that: while compliments and affirmations are nice to hear from the people you value, you have to affirm yourself as well and cannot depend on others to validate you. You give people too much power when you allow them to control your self-worth and when you rely on their opinions to validate you. You have to be in a mindset that even if nobody compliments you or tells you how amazing you are, you know your worth and you are fine with affirming yourself. Affirmations are important to recite to yourself. More importantly, you have to believe what God says about you over people's opinions. The closer your relationship is to The Lord, the more you learn about yourself.

I knew the relationship was over when he tried to pretend as though he would be too busy to spend time with me on my birthday. He behaved as if it would be a burden for him to make plans. This was quite the switch up because initially, he brought it to my attention that we would have to celebrate my birthday either a week before or after because he would be attending a conference out of town. Anyone who knows me knows that I am big on birthdays, so this was definitely a deal breaker. In addition to his nonchalant attitude, his communication efforts with me were beginning to become nonexistent. He was already distancing himself and used the excuse of being too tired to return phone calls and text messages. I knew all too well what that meant and frankly, I was tired of feeling inadequate and being treated less than what I deserved.

Finally, I made the decision to end it. I tried to call that morning and still no answer after three days. Enough was enough. I had to make my move while I had enough strength and thus, I was left with no choice but to send him a text that read, "I'm sorry but I can no longer be in this relationship, God Bless."

He responded "I feel the same way."

As relieved as I was that it was over, I was also disappointed. "Why does this always happen to me?" I thought. "I get so close to being married and having a family and it never works out." I began to question everything. — *Am I called to singleness? Do I really know the difference between the voice of God and my own? What is wrong with me? Why does it seem that everyone else is married but me?* — I felt so humiliated. I really had hoped it would work out. Looking back, I am glad the relationship ended and did not progress to marriage. I would have been miserable trying to be who he wanted me to be and I would have completely forfeited my destiny. Eventually, I found the 'good' in goodbye.

What I learned from this experience was invaluable. It taught me that I could actually date someone in holiness and not engage in fornication. It also taught me that I could have avoided all of this if I would have been obedient to wise counsel. You see, I sought godly wise counsel and actually ended the relationship with him. We both agreed to just remain friends and because I ended it, he wanted to get to know me even more. I thought I could handle being friends but eventually, emotions got invested and my spirit got cloudy. Because of this, I decided to go against wise counsel and enter into a relationship with him. My emotions had me thinking I was doing the right thing but spiritually I was all wrong and out of order.

Deep down inside, although I initially verbally ended it, I was still rather intrigued of what it would be like to be with him. I was not at a mature state or strong enough to just be friends.

If I had a chance to talk to the 'me' back then I would say: just keep pursuing God until you have a full understating of who you are in him. Focus on your purpose and His will for your life. The rest will come in due season.

6

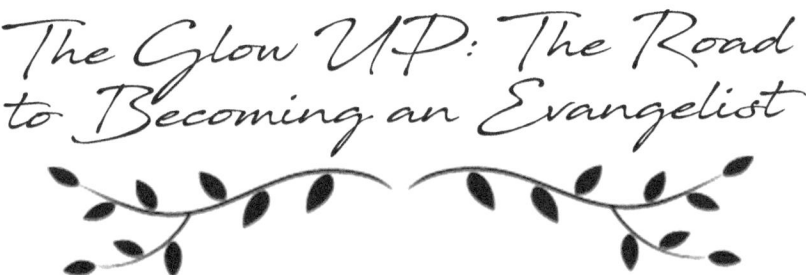
The Glow UP: The Road to Becoming an Evangelist

> *"And he gave some, apostles; and some, prophets; and some, evangelists; and some, pastors and teachers; For the perfecting of the saints, for the work of the ministry, for the edifying of the body of Christ..."* **Ephesians 4:11-12**

Who would have thought that the little girl that was quiet and shy, that grew up in subsidized housing in a single parent household, and was stereotypically in danger of becoming a statistic; would be chosen by God to be called into ministry.

We all wait for that moment in life when we can finally look at our past and laugh; when we can finally look in the mirror, smile, and be proud of who we are and all we have accomplished. That moment when all the things that made us different or set apart are now actually working in our favor; where we have finally grown into our big eyes or forehead, where we finally feel comfortable enough to show off our "chicken legs" or aren't afraid to go to the beach and wear a two piece, even if we are not 'Sport's Illustrated' ready. This, my friends, is what I call the **"Glow Up."**

Now, *Glowing Up* does not happen overnight; it can take years. It is a blossoming and a becoming. It is an awakening of knowing and loving yourself to a level in which it does not matter what anyone else thinks. You know who and whose you are. It took me almost 30 years to get to a place where I was finally happy with my life and who I was and still am becoming.

I had been searching for a church home for so many years and would always end up disappointed or disheartened because I just could not find a place that felt safe and felt like home. I was in and out of church my whole life so technically, I did not grow up in church. But the times I did spend in church, I enjoyed it.

I remember one season where we had spent at least 6 months in the church. I recall the pastor, after preaching his sermon, asking if there was anyone who wanted to be baptized. As he was explaining baptism, I thought, *I want to be closer to God and if this is going to make me closer to Him then I'm in.* I walked down the church aisle to the church altar. I was 8 years old when I made that decision.

When someone asks me when I first got saved, I say that day because that was the day I accepted Jesus as my Lord and Savior and wanted to live for Him. Jesus said in Matthew 19:14 (NKJV) *"Let the little children come to Me, and do not forbid them; for of such is the kingdom of heaven."* Jesus also said that whosoever humble themselves like as little children, the same is the greatest in the kingdom of heaven. This lets me know that when I made that decision to get baptized at the tender age of 8, I was already saved. I also count that day because when I decided to get baptized, nobody forced me or pressured me, I just wanted to be right with my Savior.

    My mom and the congregation were so shocked to see me walk to the altar. I could tell by the gasps and the applause but I couldn't understand why they were so surprised. It was not a hard decision, I wanted more of God. In retrospect, surrendering to God at age 8 is much less complicated than at age 29. Now I get it. I completely understand their gasps and excitement. They were probably thinking, *wow, what a mature decision to make as a child and to be so confident in The Lord.* Even though I strayed away from the house of The Lord as I got older, I still had some type of relationship. There were moments where I would pray and listen to gospel music; and I attended church on Christmas and Resurrection Sunday. And though I was not in church on a consistent basis, some days I would still try to catch the church van that came to my neighborhood.

    My journey from that day until now was not what one would call a typical "minister's story" you may hear about growing up in the church. Regardless, I know that even in my peaks and valleys, God was with me every step and knew that eventually I would rededicate my life to Him just as I did on that day.

Even in my wilderness experience, whenever I would try to go too far left, the Holy Spirit would convict me. I remember going through bouts of abstinence in relationships because I would feel so convicted about having sex before marriage. This would only cause tension in my relationships resulting in me giving in or the relationship ending.

THEY THAT SOW IN TEARS SHALL REAP IN JOY

I will always remember my first time visiting my now church, *Liberation Church International*. As soon as I walked through the doors of the church I felt at home. My friend had invited me the day before to come. The next day I got there early not realizing that intercessory prayer would be happening. One of the ministers was leading prayer and as he began to pray I felt the tangible presence of the Holy Spirit. I felt an indescribable sensation, something that I never felt before. It was a supernatural experience for sure. As I was touched by the Spirit I began to cry. Out of concern, my friend asked if I was ok. I nodded yes.

At the time, I did not understand why I was crying. But now, as I reflect, they were tears of joy. Why? Because I knew my prayers had been answered. For years, I prayed for a church home...*years*. I tried other churches but as I stated before, I just never fit in. I also believed that healing and transformation was taking place in that moment. I was no longer shy about praising the Lord during praise and worship. After losing my beloved brother and letting go of a 4 year relationship, I was thankful for what God had brought me through. After months of being depressed, worried, anxious, and experiencing so many losses; I was finally experiencing joy!

Even after that supernatural experience, I was still hesitant to join. I was afraid because I knew joining a church that was so powerful would change my life forever. It took me about three weeks to make my decision. When the invitation came to join, I was the first one to come to the altar. I cried because a huge weight was lifted off of my shoulders.

Then came even more confirmation that I was at home. It was an embrace that I had with my First Lady that spoke volumes. She gave me a hug and a kiss on the cheek. This was confirmation because my brother who passed away would do the same thing to people he met to comfort them. He would give them a big hug and a kiss on the cheek and say, "I love you". I believe that was God's way of comforting me and letting me know I was in the right place and that I made the right decision.

It did not take long for me to get acclimated and I started serving not too long after I joined. I wanted to help carry out the vision and help wherever was needed the most. It seemed the biggest need at the time was our Family & Friends Day. This is a day where family and friends are encouraged to join us in service & fellowship with us. So my first assignment was to coordinate the Family and Friends Day event. I honestly did not feel qualified to do this. My first thought was, *Oh no I'm going to let them down, they must have made a mistake, I don't think I can do this.* It took a lot of prayer to execute this assignment because I had to do things out of my comfort zone such as call and communicate with men.

I always felt uncomfortable around men. Part of it was because of the events that happened to me when I was younger and part of it was because I did not grow up in a house with both parents. For the longest time, I struggled to look my Spiritual Father in the eye because I was insecure about interacting with men. On top of that, I had to get in front of the whole church to make an announcement about Family and Friends Day. This was a big deal for me. I never had to talk in front of a congregation before and I felt so uncomfortable but I got through it.

The Family & Friends Day was successful even though there was a slight mishap. Somehow the power went out and the moon bounce deflated while kids were in it. Since then, I have always made sure to have a generator on hand. I can now laugh at what happened that day, but at the time, I was devastated. My anxiety was at an all-time high after that incident and I was afraid it ruined the kid's experience. But they couldn't have cared less. They thought it was all fun and as a matter of fact, my mother and I had to pull them out of the moon bounce because they were still trying to stay in as it was tumbling down.

We did not run out of food, everyone enjoyed their self, and we had great attendance. Through it all, I learned that I was capable of more than I thought. Perhaps that is why my pastor chose me to be the coordinator; to stir up my strengths and increase my confidence in carrying out an assignment.

In that season, I fully engulfed myself in the things of God. I underwent a spiritual boot camp, if you will. I exercised in godliness through various activities such as serving on different ministries, spending a lot of time in prayer, studying His Word, and so much more. I became the leader of the praise dance ministry, a part of the pastoral care ministry, as well as various committees.

I went from not having much of a prayer life to praying corporately every Monday and Friday. This season was my training ground. God was preparing me for something, I just did not know what at the time, but I just was obedient and put my trust and faith in Him. I was more focused on my relationship with God more than anything else. The Bible says God is a rewarder of those who diligently seek Him. My reward was that God redeemed the time. There was a supernatural acceleration that took place and to this day I am in awe of God's work. In 2013, I joined the church; and by 2015, I became an Evangelist.

BECOMING AN EVANGELIST

In the middle of all that was going on with the back and forth of the relationship between myself and the pastor mentioned in the chapter *Contoured*, I was preparing for one of the most important decisions I had ever made. I had said 'yes' to the call of ministry and was preparing spiritually for the office of an Evangelist. I now understand the saying "the anointing costs you something."

Initially, I was only supposed to be in the class for six months because that was the requirement for my role as an armor bearer. I had no intentions of being a minister or preacher. It was not until I began to attend the classes that I felt God calling me to more. Although I did not understand it, I was willing to submit to the process. I figured as long as I showed up to the trainings and stayed faithful, God would take care of the rest. But it was not easy at all.

During my season of grief and loss, if someone would have told me at the time that God would lead me to a church where I would grow spiritually and become an Evangelist, I would have laughed and thought, *that person must not be in their right mind.* I could not see myself through God's eyes. In my mind, I did not have the credentials to be a minister. I did not grow up on a pew nor come from a long history of pastors or preachers. I was not comfortable with speaking the Word of God in public, I was not comfortable with praying in front of others, I was afraid of the microphone, and I could barely get through the announcements.

"How was God going to use someone like me to spread the Gospel?" I thought. He prepared me in His own way.

One of my first assignments, that I now realize was training me, was when I was asked by my co-pastor — affectionately known as First Lady — to lead a workshop titled "Your Body is a Temple."

I get asked all the time, "How did you know you were an Evangelist?" To simply put it, God told me. However, it was a process that began during my church's anniversary celebration. After the preacher finished preaching he began to prophesy over me. I wrote the prophecy down.

The Lord used him to tell me this:

> "Some things happen because of you, some circumstances you didn't ask for. By this time, you expected to accomplish certain things but the harder you try the harder it gets away. The Lord says I'm going to redeem the time, it's going to be a year of acceleration. Things are going to start falling into place. It's going to work this time!"

At the time of that word, I was 30 and single. I just knew by 25 I would be married with kids. However, that was not my story. Upon hearing the prophecy my immediate thought was "Wow!" "This is the year it is going to happen for me! I'm going to be a wife and a mother. It's really going to happen!!!"

I was so excited that I did not even consider praying on that word for more understanding and clarity. Still a little immature in the area of understanding prophecy, I didn't know that sometimes the manifestation is not always what you thought it would look like. I have since grown to know that I have to dig deeper when a prophetic word comes forth and seek the face of God through fasting and prayer. Because I held on to this notion, I entertained the relationship I discussed in the previous chapter. He fit part of the description being a pastor and all. Even though he was not my type, I still dated him with high hopes that we would get married soon. I also put up with a lot of things that I should not have and ignored all of the warning signs for the sake of thinking he was the one. Interestingly enough, dating him made me seek the face of God even more in regards to my purpose and what God was trying to do with me. So in spite of everything, it all eventually worked for my good and provoked me to be the bold and confident woman that I am today.

Now I have an understanding of what that prophetic word was talking about. God was speaking to me though the Prophet about how He was going to prosper me spiritually. That the longing and desire I had to know Christ on a more intimate level was finally going to happen. I was so caught up in my carnal desires that I almost missed the move of God. I'm so glad that I was surrounded by people to remind me of who I was when I was in that relationship.

Understand that pursuing purpose is not always easy. There are times when it feels like you are sacrificing everything, like the things you believe brings you happiness or what you believe is the right solution for your life. Many are called but few are chosen. I chose purpose with every fiber of my being. I chose purpose with tears and trembles. I chose purpose with fear and uncertainty. Then finally I chose purpose with love and boldness.

REMOVING THE FIG LEAVES

I used to go around in life trying to hide my pain and suffering. I would bury my emotions and hide behind the façade that I "had it altogether". I would pretend as though things did not bother me when they really did. I would hold grudges and hide behind anger as my shields. I hid behind shyness, insecurity, and low self-esteem because I became comfortable with a false identity. The truth was I wanted to come out of hiding to remove the fig leaves and be free to yield to God's plan for my life. It was hard to embrace my God given identity. It was uncomfortable and felt very awkward the times I would try.

I remember being asked to do the announcements for my church. This was something I initially turned down because I did not want to stand in front of people. What if I said the wrong thing? I felt I was not worthy to stand behind a podium. Plus, I was new and I did not feel comfortable enough to do it but eventually, I gave in and did it anyway.

I remember the first time. I started off well and then it all went downhill. I could not stop trembling and was so afraid that my hand was shaking. After it was over, people encouraged me but I was so embarrassed. I would rehearse days before and even practice what I would say and still the same thing would happen every time. It did not matter how much time I spent in preparation, I would still get nervous and sometimes anxious about doing the announcements. Then one day I finally had a breakthrough moment. After six months of doing them, I began to get better. I began to get more confident and I started to relax and be myself. I realized that I did not have to hide me or be stiff. If I just relaxed and did not put so much pressure on myself to be perfect, the situation would be less tense. Eventually I grew to the point where I no longer needed to spend hours rehearsing the announcements and I did not panic if there were any last minute changes.

After that, I was challenged again. One day out of nowhere my Pastor/First Lady/spiritual mother called me. She said she had been praying and seeking The Lord regarding our women's conference. She wanted me to teach a Gospel Zumba class and then facilitate a workshop. Since I was a health and wellness coach, she wanted me to discuss the body being a temple.

My immediate response was, "You know I don't talk that much."

She laughed and said, "I know but you'll be fine."

So, I agreed to do it. She gave me a month's notice and I spent the next 30 days really seeking the face of God. I had never done this before. I needed revelation and I needed to see beyond the text as my spiritual father would say.

I meditated on the verse that says "your body is a temple" and I thought, *what, exactly, is a temple?* I remember the story in the Bible about Solomon building a temple for the Arc of the Covenant. As I began to study the process in which it took for him to build the first temple, I learned how King Solomon used real material and nothing artificial. People sacrificed and gave precious jewels for the construction of the temple and so much detail was put into it. The whole process took 7 years to complete and after it was completed the Glory fell so thickly that the Priests could not even perform service.

It was in that time that what The Lord was showing me about me, was true. He was birthing the preacher inside of me and using this platform at the women's conference as my first assignment. In the days leading up to the conference, God would give me more revelation about the body being a temple and gave me great insight on how the construction of King Solomon's temple is relative to how we take care of our temple while we are here on earth. God showed me beyond the text and revealed His mysteries to me. This was truly a faith-walk for me as I had never did anything like this before in my life.

When the day had finally come, I was not so much nervous but excited. I was excited to share and teach on what God showed me but before I did the workshop (and talk for 45 minutes), I had to teach the Gospel Zumba class.

While rehearsing for Gospel Zumba days leading up to the conference, I was so focused on perfecting the moves of the workout and making sure I choreographed a good class, that I did not even think about the spiritual side of Gospel Zumba.

That women's conference was the first time I ever taught a Gospel Zumba class. Gospel Zumba and regular Zumba are two different things and I was used to teaching Zumba which included songs of various genres such as Latin, hip hop, reggae and more. But Gospel Zumba was a completely different class. I felt more like I was leading a praise session rather than teaching a Gospel Zumba class. What happened next was something I did not even consider when preparing for the class. The Glory fell, people started to worship and shout, and some could not even finish doing the workout.

For a moment, I was just frozen and in awe of the move of God. Humbled that God would chose to use me in this capacity. Then I realized, I was in divine alignment. All that I had gone through in the past before rededicating my life to Christ was for this moment. When the class was over one of the visitors came up to me and said, "God's gonna use you!"

I thought to myself, "Wow, really?!?" I never thought of being used by God. I did not think I had enough of Him in me to be used by Him. I thought it took years after you rededicate your life to Christ to get to a point where He trusts you enough to use you. What she said it stuck with me throughout my entire process of becoming an Evangelist.

After the Gospel Zumba class, it was time to teach on the body being a temple. By the grace of God, I had enough content to talk for 45 minutes. In that 45 minutes I was able to give conference attendees practical as well as spiritual ways to take care of their temple.

Finally, I felt like I was living and walking in purpose. I no longer felt lost. For the first time in my life I had clear and distinct direction on what I was created to do.

Later on, during the meet and greet at the conference's evening service, I saw one of the attendees and gave her a hug. Once we embraced, she whispered in my ear and said "You Saved My Life." I was blown away again! I was so caught up in the moment, I did not have a response and I did not ask her to elaborate. God was sending confirmation throughout the day.

Later on that night, I thought about what she said and the visions God showed me. *Maybe God does want to use me to help save people.* I was still not sure how He wanted to use me and there were still some doubts. I did not think being in ministry was something God wanted for my life and I certainly did not think He would call me to preach, so I ruled myself out.

But He did.

This was never a part of my plan nor was it something I could even have imagined. As I reflected on those times of obscurity about my calling, I was reminded that His ways are not my ways and His thoughts are not my thoughts. Because I listened to God and served in the capacity of an armor bearer, even though I did not feel qualified, that act of obedience positioned me to have to attend Minister in Training (MIT) class. The MIT class was a requirement for armor bearers. Had it not been a requirement for armor bearers to be in the class I would have never even considered attending MIT.

If at any time of your life you are unsure about what your purpose is or what it is God has called you to do, you'll find peace when you start to embrace the steps that lead you to your destination. Obeying God's instructions will always set you on the right path.

My transition from being a minister in training to an Evangelist had a few unexpected bumps in the road. I went through the awkward stage of "where do I fit in now?". With any elevation, there is a sacrifice required of you. The hardest thing for me was being ok with everyone not being happy for me and still being able to love them. I had to learn how to not let my emotions supersede my godliness. It was hard for me to adjust to the fact that because now I had a title people began to treat me differently. Some were intimidated and some were just plain jealous. If only they knew my story and the hell I went through; and the work and sacrifice it took. This was not something that I intentionally planned, this was something that God designed for me. I could not understand why everyone around me was not happy and I did not understand where all the animosity was coming from.

    At the time, I did not understand it, but I get it now. God always has a way of bringing things to light and removing people who were never meant to stay in your life in the first place. With promotion sometimes comes pain but also peace. The pain is from the way others will treat you because now they somehow perceive you as a threat or an enemy and peace from knowing you are in the will of God regardless of the reactions of other people.

    My first year in ministry was very stressful because I put so much pressure on myself to be perfect. I did not want to make a mistake or disappoint anyone. It was also lonely at times in a sense that it was hard to express how I was feeling. No one verbally told me to my face that they had some type of animosity against me but when you are a spiritual person you can feel things without people having to say it to your face. I felt the shift in attitudes and I could tell there were undercover conversations being had. I learned that people will manifest their true feelings in two types of situations: **when you are at rock bottom and when you are prospering.** In my case, the position in which I was elevated to revealed all too well who truly had my back and was in my corner.

That season matured me and since then I have learned to not be distracted by the actions, intentions or attitudes of others but to have compassion. Underneath someone's jealousy or envy is actually an admirer that may lack the understanding of how to truly celebrate the successes of others.

7

Showing Up

There is so much required of me these days and I am so thankful to God for it. I am an Evangelist, a health and wellness coach, Zumba instructor, a mentor, an entrepreneur, a writer/author, an innovative product creator and so much more.

It is my purpose in life to help people reach their destination and God given purpose. I believe God uses me as a bridge to help people get to their next place in life. I can confidently say my truth and purpose now, but there was a time I was afraid to show up.

One of the hardest things sometimes is saying who we are and what our purpose is. I challenge you to not make the mistake that I did for so many years. I used to hide who I really was because I had a tough time balancing humility and confidence. Whatever God designed you to be, be that authentically and don't be ashamed. It is never prideful or boastful to be who God designed you to be. I believe it is a slap in the face to hide who you are and to hide what God created you to do. You actually do a disservice to others when you don't show up because somebody needs the gifts and the talents you have. They need to hear your voice and your message. So don't be afraid to not only show up, but show out. The world is waiting on you and somebody has a need for what you have and what God has placed on the inside of you.

I know from experience that somebody needs what you have. For the longest time I struggled with whether or not to be a Zumba instructor, or being in front of people to teach, or even being a health and wellness coach. I would think, "Who is going to believe me?" I am very curvy and far from skinny. I would think who is going to take me seriously because I am curvy. However, I now realize what I thought was a disadvantage actually worked to my advantage. Because I am curvy, it actually inspired those who are not stick figures to want to work out with me and feel comfortable with working out with me.

Show up even when you do not feel like it. There are times where I had to attend business meetings and networking meetings. There were different events where I did not feel like being there. I almost did not go at all or I went and sat in the car for a few minutes and tried to talk myself out of going. Thoughts would race through my mind like, *what am I doing here, what are people going to say, what are they going to think of me, how are they going to react, is this a waste of time* or *what's the point of being here?* Every time I did not give into my negative thinking or did not give into talking myself out of not showing up, I was tremendously blessed. I would receive invitations to teach Zumba or different business opportunities.

There have been events I went to where I did not feel my best self because of various circumstances going on in my life. There were some times I would go to events and I was crying on the inside because of what was going on in my life. I did not want to be around people at all. What kept me from staying in the house and having a pity party was telling myself that I have to get through this moment. I had to realize that the situation I am in now will pass. When I got through that moment, on the other side was opportunity and success.

SHOW UP FOR OTHERS

How many times have you invited someone somewhere because you needed them there for support but you were not sure if they would come through? But the moment you look out to see if they are there and you laid eyes on them, you got a second wind or an extra boost of confidence. That same feeling you got from someone being there for you is the same sensation others will feel when they invite you somewhere and you actually commit to being there. It does not matter how big or small the event may be. If somebody took that step to invite you and took the time out to ask you to be there for them nine times out of ten, they actually want you to be there.

When you take the time to show your friends, family, loved ones, colleagues or whoever is in your circle that you will be there for them, they will usually show the same courtesy. This is how support systems are built. No matter what anyone else says, we all need support systems. Iron sharpens iron. We cannot accomplish our visions and dreams alone, we need people to help us run with it.

To show up means you are not ashamed of who you are and you understand that you do not need to apologize for being great.

8

Naked and Not Ashamed

In the chapter, Body Love, I discussed feeling naked even though I was fully clothed. Which makes me pose the question: *what do you do when you feel naked but you are fully clothed?* Do you add more layers to try and cover up your shame or your past even more, or do you redefine it? I have come to know that adding more layers only perpetuates the underlying issues you try to cover up. Eventually, what you try to hide will peep through every artificial layer and come to the surface of truth, your truth. It is only then where God gives us the grace and mercy to redefine our nakedness instead of trying to hide who we are and what we have been through.

Naked and Not Ashamed 111

Instead of allowing my past to hold me in bondage and keep me from being free, I decided to write this memoir and not be ashamed but to bare it all. To reveal all of my truth; the shameful and humiliating experiences I endured, the times of disappointment and achievement; to empower others to live a life in which God originally intended. God never wanted us to live a life where we felt like we could not be everything He called us to be. Life and all of its twists and turns can have a way of dimming our light, but God wants our light to shine.

When Adam and Eve realized they were naked because of the sin they committed, they tried to fix their sinful nakedness by covering themselves up with fig leaves. The fig leaves only fixed the symptom but did not solve the real issue. The fig leaves were only a temporary solution to a much deeper problem. Fig leaves can represent anything we use to cover up our past. Whether those are embarrassing and painful experiences, past mistakes, or past failures. We may use appearances such as clothes, fashion, cars, and money to cover up our nakedness. We even may use make-up, people pleasing, over achieving, and bad habits to hide our truth.

These types of fig leaves cannot sustain us forever. There will always be some type of voided feeling and a desire to be free. At some point you will have to remove the fig leaves and work your way back to a place of restoration; the way God originally intended all of us to be which was **naked and not ashamed.**

About the Author

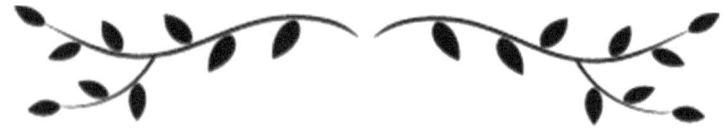

Kia Potts is a Richmond, VA native. She is the author of *Eating Healthy on the Go: A Restaurant Dining Guide for the Busy Person on the Move* and the creator of *A Better You Confidence Course.* She is an Evangelist, Health and Wellness Coach, Motivational Speaker and Licensed Zumba Instructor. She has been featured on the Sharvette Mitchell Radio Show, Speak to Your Spirit Radio Show, and Empowering Hope Radio Show. Kia has also appeared on CBS Virginia This Morning as well as in the pages of The Richmond Times Dispatch.

It is her belief that people establish well-balanced, wealthy lives by first living a healthy lifestyle and in order to truly prosper in life one must constantly strive to improve the status of their mental, physical, emotional, and spiritual health. It is her passion and purpose in life to be a bridge for those seeking and desiring to live a healthy wealthy lifestyle.

Kia holds a Master's Degree in Public Health. She is active in her community and church. Spending quality time with family and friends is what brings balance to her busy lifestyle. When her adventurous side kicks in, she enjoys traveling, restaurant hopping, taking trendy fitness classes, obstacle courses and spontaneous weekend getaways.

iamkiapotts.com | @iamkiapotts

www.ingramcontent.com/pod-product-compliance
Lightning Source LLC
Chambersburg PA
CBHW021132300426
44113CB00006B/393